T0195110

GENERAL MEDICAL KNOWLEDGE FOR FOR EYECARE PARAPROFESSIONALS

GENERAL MEDICAL KNOWLEDGE FOR EYECARE PARAPROFESSIONALS

Marvin Bittinger, MD

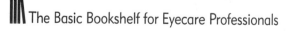 The Basic Bookshelf for Eyecare Professionals

Series Editors: Janice K. Ledford, COMT • Ken Daniels, OD • Robert Campbell, MD

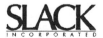 6900 Grove Road, Thorofare, NJ 08086

Publisher: John H. Bond
Editorial Director: Amy E. Drummond
Assistant Editor: Lauren Biddle

Copyright © 1999 by SLACK Incorporated

All rights reserved. No part of this book may be reproduced, stored in a retrieval system or transmitted in any form or by any means, electronic, mechanical, photocopying, recording or otherwise, without written permission from the publisher, except for brief quotations embodied in critical articles and reviews.

Bittinger, Marvin
    General medical knowledge for eyecare paraprofessionals/Marvin Bittinger
        p. cm. — (The Basic Bookshelf for Eyecare Professionals)
        Includes bibliographical references and index.
        ISBN 1-55642-334-9 (alk. paper)
        1. Internal medicine. 2. Medical sciences. 3. Eye—Diseases.
    4. Ophthalmic assistants. 5. Optometric assistants. 6. Ocular manifestations
    of general diseases. I. Title. II. Series.
        [DNLM: 1. Medicine. 2. Eye manifestations. 3. Ophthalmic assistants.
    WB 100 B6172g 1998]
    RC48.B49   1998
    616—DC21
    DNLM/DLC
    for Library of Congress   98-21940
                                                                                                CIP

Published by: SLACK Incorporated
                  6900 Grove Road
                  Thorofare, NJ 08086-9447 USA
                  Telephone: 609-848-1000
                  Fax: 609-853-5991
                  World Wide Web: http://www.slackinc.com

Contact SLACK Incorporated for more information about other books in this field or about the availability of our books from distributors outside the United States.

Authorization to photocopy items for internal or personal use, or the internal or personal use of specific clients, is granted by SLACK Incorporated, provided that the appropriate fee is paid directly to Copyright Clearance Center, 222 Rosewood Drive, Danvers, MA 01923 USA, 978-750-8400. Prior to photocopying items for educational classroom use, please contact the CCC at the address above. Please reference Account Number 9106324 for SLACK Incorporated's Professional Book Division.

For further information on CCC, check CCC Online at the following address: http://www.copyright.com.

Last digit is print number: 10 9 8 7 6 5 4 3 2 1

Contents

Acknowledgments

Thanks to my wife, Brenda, for giving up her time for me to use while writing this book; to Jan Ledford for giving me the opportunity to write it; to James Talmadge for helping illustrate it; and to Jan Gray for keeping me going when I wanted to quit.

About the Author

Dr. Bittinger received a BA degree from Asbury College in Wilmore, KY in 1971. In 1974, he received his MD degree from the University of Tennessee. He is board certified in emergency medicine, and for the last 2 years has served as medical director for Eyesight Associates, a 10-office eyecare practice in central Georgia. He is married and has two daughters.

Introduction

The human body is a uniquely designed "earth suit" allowing us to work in, and relate to, the hostile environment of Earth. It is by far the most complex and fascinating of living organisms. Thousands of hours and millions of dollars are spent annually exploring the intricacies of its structure and function. Obviously, I can barely scratch the surface of bodily understanding in the following chapters. Thus, my goal is to present the basic concepts of anatomy and physiology as well as an overview of common diseases. I believe this will provide a solid foundation in general medical knowledge for those working as eyecare professionals.

What The Patient Needs To Know

- Your body is a collection of systems that work together. Because of this, any disease or condition you have may also affect your eyes.

- Do not ignore eye symptoms because you think they are normal for someone with your condition.

- Any time your regular doctor diagnoses a new condition, be sure to tell your eyecare practitioner.

- Just because you have a disease or condition, it does not mean you will experience the eye problems associated with it.

- Always keep your appointments for eye exams and follow-ups. Early detection is often the key in preventing severe problems.

The Study Icons

The *Basic Bookshelf for Eyecare Professionals* is quality educational material designed for professionals in all branches of eyecare. Because so many of you want to expand your careers, we have made a special effort to include information needed for certification exams. When these study icons appear in the margin of a *Series* book, it is your cue that the material next to the icon (which may be a paragraph or an entire section) is listed as a criteria item for a certification examination. Please use this key to identify the appropriate icon:

OptA   optometric assistant

OptT   optometric technician

OphA   ophthalmic assistant

OphT   ophthalmic technician

OphMT   ophthalmic medical technologist

LV   low vision subspecialty

Srg   ophthalmic surgical assisting subspecialty

CL   contact lens registry

Optn   opticianry

RA   retinal angiographer

Chapter 1

The Body as a Whole

OptT

OptA

KEY POINTS

- The body has four basic parts: cells, tissues, organs, and organ systems.

- The major systems of the body are musculoskeletal, nervous, gastrointestinal, respiratory, cardiovascular, genitourinary, and reproductive.

- The three regions of the body are head and neck, trunk, and limbs.

Basic Structure of the Body

The body is composed of four basic parts: cells, tissues, organs, and organ systems. Everything in the body is associated with one of these four basic parts.

The simplest of these are cells. Cells provide the structural framework for all other elements of the body. They are the smallest division of the body that can reproduce and perform metabolic functions. Each cell specializes in performing specific functions. For example, muscle cells contract and cause an arm to move, and skin cells form a protective shield that prevents harmful bacteria from invading the body.

Cells that perform similar functions are grouped together to form tissues. Combining like functioning cells greatly increases the amount of work that can be done. Individually, nerve cells can accomplish very little. Grouping many nerve cells together enables them to transmit electrical impulses that direct thinking, feeling, and motion.

When two or more tissues are combined, they form an organ. While tissues allow more work to be done, merging tissues into organs permits specific types of work to be accomplished. The heart, for example, is a combination of several tissues that work in concert to pump blood to all parts of the body. No one tissue could do this alone.

Finally, organ systems are an alliance of multiple organs that perform many functions to benefit the entire body. The esophagus, stomach, intestines, and other organs form the digestive system which, through multiple processes, breaks down food to provide energy for the body.

The organ systems are connected together and coordinated to form the body as a whole.

Body Parts and Functions

Like steel girders in a tall building, the bones form the superstructure that gives shape and strength to the body. When bones surround vital organs, as does the skull, they provide protection from external trauma. The bones are held together by fibrous bands called ligaments. Joints lie between the bones, and allow for movement and flexibility. There are 206 bones in the body.

The muscles produce the movement of the body. They are attached to bones via dense cords of connective tissue called tendons. These attachments allow the muscles to exert leverage across joints and produce motion.

Movement must be controlled and coordinated to be useful. The nervous system performs this function. The brain is the central processing unit for the body. Input is received by the brain from the five senses (touch, smell, sight, hearing, and taste), as well as a myriad of other sensors all over the body. Once the information is processed, the brain sends instructions to the body via the spinal cord and peripheral nerves.

The activities of the body require energy. The digestive system converts food into fuel that can be used by cells to produce energy. Food is taken into the mouth, broken up by chewing, and swallowed. The esophagus transports the food to the stomach where chemicals are added to further break down the food. From the stomach, the food passes into the intestines where enzymes are added, and energy-producing nutrients are absorbed into the bloodstream. The nutrients are taken to the cells where they are transformed into energy by a process called metabolism.

Cellular metabolism requires oxygen. The oxygen required to produce energy is extracted from the air by the lungs. Inhaled air is transported to the lungs by the trachea and bronchial tubes. Here the air is collected in small sacs called alveoli, where the oxygen is separated and diffused into the bloodstream. The oxygen is then carried to the cells by the blood.

Transportation within the body is provided by blood and the heart. Blood exists in virtually every tissue of the body. Nutrients, oxygen, and waste products are picked up and delivered to various destinations in the body by the blood. Its movement is caused by the pumping action of the heart.

The kidneys, lungs, and intestines compose the body's waste disposal team. The kidneys filter the blood, removing liquid waste. After extracting nutrients from food passing through them, the intestines expel the leftover solid waste through the rectum. The lungs handle the gaseous waste product of metabolism, carbon dioxide. When we exhale, this gas leaves the lungs, and is vented into the atmosphere.

As death is a certainty for all bodies, the reproductive system insures the survival of the human species by forming new human bodies. Once conceived, the forming child is nurtured within the uterus until mature enough to survive in the outside world. Then, at birth, uterine contractions expel the child through the cervix and vagina.

Regions of the Body

The body is divided into three regions: the head and neck, trunk, and limbs (Figure 1-1).

Head and Neck

The head and neck occupy the uppermost part of the body. The head houses the brain, which is the body's computer control center. Virtually all bodily functions and actions begin in, and are directed by, the brain. The neck contains a number of large blood vessels, such as the carotid arteries, which are the main blood supply of the brain. Also contained in the neck are the esophagus, which transfers food from the mouth to the stomach, and the trachea, which carries air from the mouth and nose to the lungs. Two major glands are also located in the neck— the thyroid gland and the parathyroid gland.

Trunk

The trunk is the largest region of the body. It extends from the base of the neck to the area where the legs join the pelvic bone. With the exception of the brain, all the body's vital organs are housed in the trunk. The trunk is divided into three areas.

Thorax

The base of the neck and the diaphragm form the upper and lower limits of the thorax. Ribs and part of the spine form its lateral boundaries. It contains two very important organs— the heart and the lungs.

Abdomen

The abdomen lies between the thorax and the pelvis. The upper border is the diaphragm, while the lower border is the pelvis. It contains organs of digestion, including the stomach and intestines, as well as organs of excretion, such as the kidneys. The liver, spleen, and adrenal glands are also housed in the abdomen.

Pelvis

The pelvis is the part of the trunk contained within the bounds of the pelvic bone. Its primary contents are the bladder and reproductive organs.

Limbs

The third region of the body is the limbs— the arms and legs. They give us the ability to move and accomplish meaningful tasks.

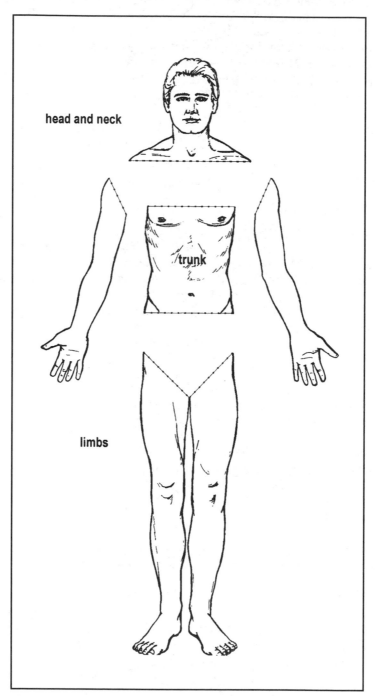

Figure 1-1. Regions of the body (Medical Illustration Library, General Anatomy One image GA1-1008; Williams and Wilkins: 1994).

Positional Terms

Like using a compass and a map to take a trip, positional terms give the ability to know position and direction when studying or treating the human body (Figure 1-2).

The anatomic position is the standard position used to describe location in the body. It is defined as standing erect, eyes looking forward to the horizon, arms by the side, palms of hands directed forward, thumbs outward, and toes directed forward.

The midline is an imaginary line drawn vertically down the middle of the body while in anatomical position. It separates the body into right and left halves.

A number of positional terms are used when describing the body. All of these are defined relative to the anatomic position.

Anterior, Ventral— Nearer the front surface of the body
Posterior, Dorsal— Nearer the back surface of the body

Superior— Nearer the top of the head
Inferior— Nearer the soles of the feet

Medial— Nearer the midline
Lateral— Farther away from the midline

Superficial— Nearer the surface
Deep— Farther away from the surface

Ipsilateral— Same side of the body
Contralateral— Opposite side of the body

Internal— Nearer the center of the body
External— Away from the center of the body

Proximal— near a specified region
Distal— farther away from a specified region

Plantar— sole of the foot
Palmar— palm of the hand

Left— to the left of the midline to a subject in anatomic position (Figure 1-3)
Right— to the right of the midline to a subject in anatomic position

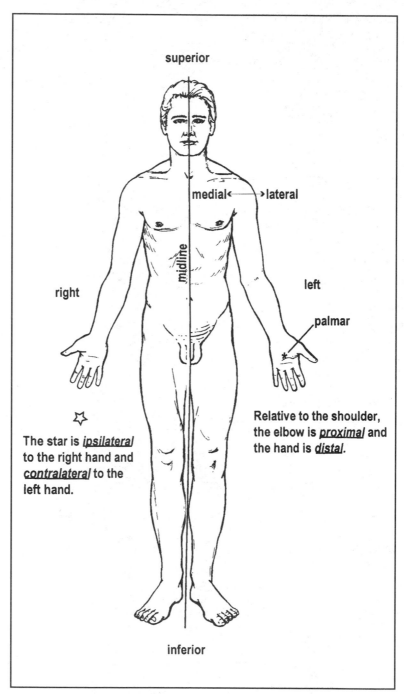

Figure 1-2. Positional terms in anatomic position (Medical Illustration Library, General Anatomy One image GA1-1008; Williams and Wilkins: 1994).

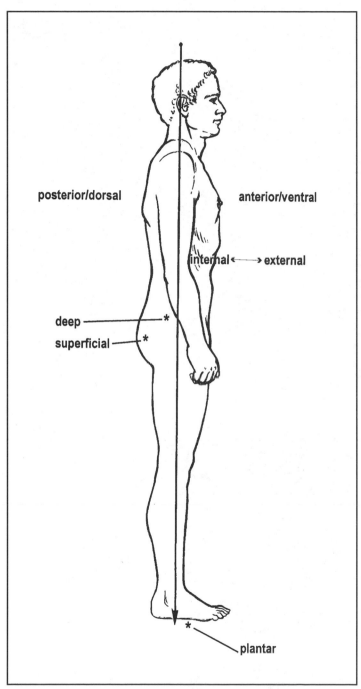

Figure 1-3. Positional terms in side view (Medical Illustration Library, General Anatomy One image GA1-1010; Williams and Wilkins: 1994).

Chapter 2

Cells and Tissues

OptT
OptA

KEY POINTS

- Cells and tissues form the basic substance of the human body.

- Organs and the systems they form derive identity and structure from their cell and tissue make-up.

- Cells are the "concrete" that the tissue "building blocks" are made from.

- Bound together, cells form the "foundation" of the human body.

Cells

The cell is the smallest living functional unit in the body. Ultimately, all medical science is based on how cells work. Diseases and their treatments originate in the structure and processes of the cell. The appearance and function of the body is the sum of cellular characteristics.

Cell Structure

Like balloons full of water, cells are thin membranes surrounding and retaining a quantity of fluid (Figure 2-1). They vary in size from 7.5 micrometers (ie, red blood cell) to 1000 micrometers (ie, ovum). Each cell is bathed in a diluted saltwater solution called tissue fluid. Cells have two major parts: the plasma membrane and the cytoplasm.

Plasma Membrane

The plasma membrane is a thin membrane (about three ten-millionths of an inch thick) that defines the outer limits of the cell. Phospholipid molecules and proteins are its main components. It has several functions.

Like the wall of a swimming pool, the plasma membrane retains the inner liquid portion of the cell. This gives each cell a distinct physical identity.

The plasma membrane serves as a gateway between fluid inside and fluid outside the cell. It determines which substances can enter the cell and which substances are kept out.

Similar to the receiver of a telephone, the plasma membrane "hears" messages from other parts of the body through protein molecules on its surface. Information received is sent to the cell interior where it is processed and acted upon.

Identifying a cell as coming from one particular individual is another of the plasma membrane's jobs. Surface molecules act as identification tags for the cell. These tags are unique to each person.

Cytoplasm

Cytoplasm is a complex fluid that fills the plasma membrane. Many important chemical reactions occur in the cytoplasm. Two groups of structures are housed in the cytoplasm: the organelles and the cytoskeleton.

Organelles are mini-organs suspended in the cytoplasm of the cell. The number and type of organelles determine individual cell function. Just like true organs, organelles carry out specific functions.

The most important organelle is the nucleus. It is usually located near the center of the cell and functions as its control center. Every other organelle is supervised by the nucleus. Located in the nucleus of human cells are 23 pairs of chromosomes. They contain about 100,000 genes that store the code that determines the make-up of each cell. The sum of cellular characteristics determines the appearance and function of the body as a whole. When a cell reproduces, the chromosomes are copied and sent to the new cell. The nucleus directs this process.

Other organelles include ribosomes, mitochondria, lysosomes, endoplasmic reticulum, golgi complex, and peroxisomes.

The cytoskeleton is a group of flexible protein fibers that form the superstructure of the cell. Their appearance is much like scaffolding used by workers to paint or repair tall buildings. Many fibers attach to the plasma membrane. This functions to give shape to the cell and to provide the cell with mechanical strength. The cytoskeleton also helps determine the distribution of organelles within the cytoplasm.

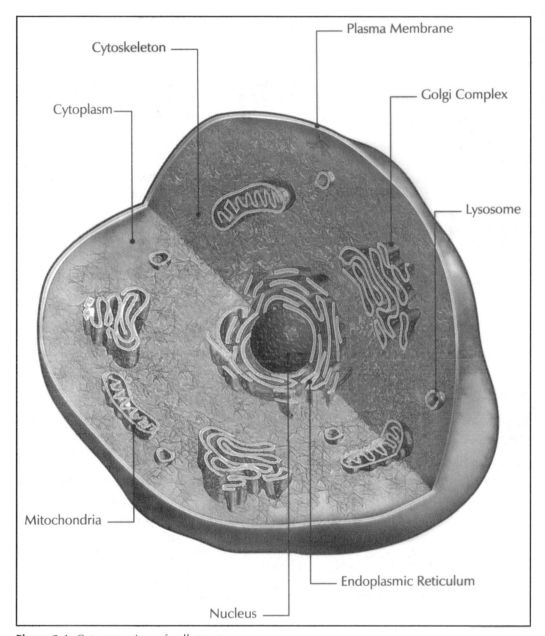

Figure 2-1. Cut away view of cell structure.

Cell Function

Cells perform all the processes necessary for life. Four activities characterize all cells:
- They produce energy
- They reproduce
- They interact with their environment
- They regulate themselves internally

Energy Production

By creating needed power, cells act as the engine of the body. Energy is produced by converting glucose and oxygen to carbon dioxide and water. This process occurs in the mitochondria, one of the cell's organelles. The chemical ATP (adenosine triphosphate) stores the energy until it is needed by the body.

Reproduction

Survival of the body depends on cell reproduction. Approximately 1% of body cells die each day. Without reproduction, we would all be dead in 100 days!

Cells divide by two processes: mitosis and cytokinesis. During mitosis, the chromosomes are copied, resulting in two identical sets. Cytokinesis, on the other hand, divides the cytoplasm in half. These two actions create two nearly identical cells.

Reproduction accomplishes three things:
- development of the body during childhood when the body is growing
- replacement of cells that die
- repair and/or replacement of cells that have been injured

External Interaction

The body is a beautiful illustration of teamwork. Each part has its function, which is carried out and coordinated with all other parts of the body. Most integration occurs at the cellular level. Cells respond in an appropriate and predictable manner to things occurring around them. For example, muscle cells respond to stimulation by electricity from nerve cells, and chemicals such as hormones alter cellular behavior. The result is a meshing of thousands of actions into an integrated whole.

Internal Regulation

Many complex chemical reactions and other processes occur in the cell. Without some type of control mechanism, chaos would result and the cell would die. Homeostasis describes the cell's ability to internally regulate itself, creating balance in the performance of its assigned functions.

Tissues

The body is composed of four types of tissues: nerve, muscle, epithelial, and connective.

Nerve Tissue

Nerve tissue is the body's postal service. It transmits messages in the form of electrical impulses from one place to another. Nerve tissue comprises the brain, the spinal cord, and the myriad of nerve fibers throughout the body.

Muscle Tissue

Movement is produced by muscle tissue. Contraction of muscles in the legs causes the body to walk. Contraction of muscle in the heart moves blood to all parts of the body. Contraction of the iris diminishes pupillary size and decreases the amount of light hitting the retina.

Epithelial Tissue

Epithelial tissue performs three functions: protection, absorption, and secretion.

Skin is the epithelial tissue with which we are most familiar. It envelops the body like a blanket, providing a protective shield against harmful elements such as bacteria.

The food we eat is processed in the digestive system. Here important nutrients are extracted and absorbed into the blood stream. Epithelial tissue, which lines the intestines, performs this function.

Salivary glands secrete saliva, which aids in the digestion of our food. Epithelial tissue is the primary tissue of salivary glands.

Connective Tissue

Connective tissue takes many different forms and is found in many different places in the body. Adipose or fat tissue insulates the body and acts as a shock absorber when trauma occurs. It also functions as a storage depot for unused energy. The connective tissue proper fills the spaces between other tissues and organs. It acts as a glue, holding bodily parts in proper position. Bone and cartilage are specialized connective tissues that give support to the body. Blood, another specialized connective tissue, is the body's transportation system, carrying nutrients and other products to all parts of the body.

Chapter 3

The Cardiovascular System

OptT

OptA

KEY POINTS

- The heart, blood vessels, and blood make up the cardiovascular system.

- Together they function as the body's transportation system.

- The cardiovascular system carries life-sustaining nutrients to all parts of the body.

Anatomy

The cardiovascular system has three divisions: central circulation, peripheral circulation, and blood.

Central Circulation

The central circulation includes the heart and surrounding blood vessels. It is the grand central station of the cardiovascular system (Figure 3-1).

The heart has long been the object of human fascination. Ancient Greeks believed it to be the seat of strength and center of physical life. Dr. William Harvey first described circulation in the 1600s.

The heart is a hollow muscle shaped like an inverted cone. It is located behind the sternum in the center of the chest. Pumping blood is its primary purpose.

Four chambers make up the inside of the heart. The right and left atria occupy the top of the heart while the right and left ventricles make up the lower part of the heart. Blood coming into the heart is received by the atria, which pump it into the ventricles. The ventricles pump blood out of the heart to the lungs and rest of the body.

Valves connect the atria and ventricles. The right atrium and right ventricle are connected by the tricuspid valve. The left atrium and left ventricle are connected by the mitral valve. When the atria pump blood into the ventricles, the valves open, allowing the blood to pass. As the ventricles contract to pump blood away from the heart, the valves close, preventing blood from re-entering the atria.

Blood is carried to and from the heart through blood vessels. These are hollow tubes made of muscle. When the muscle contracts, the vessels get smaller. Relaxation, on the other hand, makes the vessels larger. Arteries are blood vessels that carry blood away from the heart. Veins are blood vessels that carry blood to the heart.

Four major blood vessels (two veins and two arteries) connect to the heart. Blood from the lungs is transported by the pulmonary veins back to the left ventricle. The vena cava, a large vein, empties blood into the right atrium and has two parts—the superior vena cava drains blood from the upper half of the body, while the inferior vena cava carries blood from the body's lower half. The pulmonary trunk and its two branches, the right and left pulmonary arteries, move blood from the right ventricle to the lungs. The body's largest artery, the aorta, exits the left ventricle and carries blood to all parts of the body.

Two additional valves help regulate blood flow in the aorta and pulmonary trunk. The pulmonic valve is located where the pulmonary trunk exits the heart. It prevents blood from flowing back into the heart after being pumped out by the right ventricle. The aortic valve is located where the aorta leaves the heart. It prevents blood from flowing back into the heart after being pumped out by the left ventricle.

The coronary arteries supply blood to the heart muscle and branch off the aorta just as it leaves the heart. When these arteries are blocked, a heart attack results.

Blood circulates through the heart in a very organized fashion. Blood from all parts of the body comes to the right atrium via the superior and inferior venae cavae. Once in the right atrium, it is pumped through the tricuspid valve into the right ventricle. The right ventricle contracts, forcing the blood through the pulmonic valve into the pulmonary trunk. The pulmonary trunk divides into the right and left pulmonary arteries, which transfer blood to the lungs where oxygen is added. Blood from the lungs returns to the left atrium in the pulmonary veins. Contraction of the left atrium then propels blood through the mitral valve into the left ventricle. It squeezes blood past the aortic valve into the aorta, and from there to the rest of the body.

Much like electrical wiring in a house, the heart has special tissues that conduct electrical

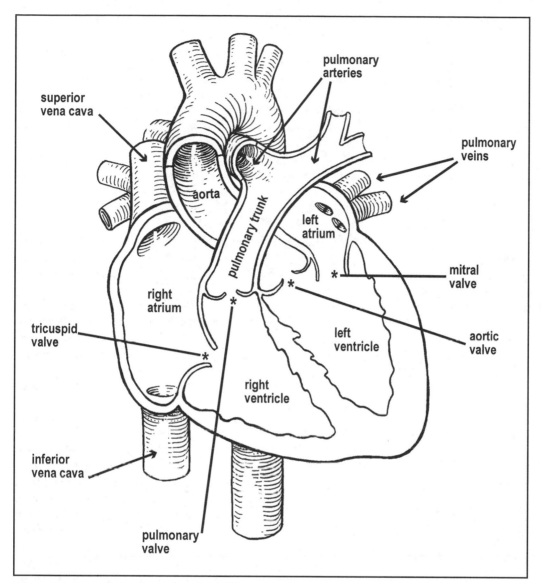

Figure 3-1. Central circulation (Medical Illustration Library, General Anatomy Two image GA2-1020; Williams and Wilkins: 1994).

impulses. These impulses cause the heart muscle to contract, resulting in blood flow. The sinoatrial (SA) node is located in the upper portion of the right atrium. This is the origin of the electricity that drives the heart. The atrioventricular (AV) node is located in the lower portion of the right atrium. It receives and transmits impulses from the SA node. A large group of fibers, called the Bundle of His, leave the AV node and divide into two branches, the right and the left bundle branches.

Peripheral Circulation

Arteries

The aorta is the largest artery in the body (about 1 inch in diameter), and is the primary source of blood flow for most other arteries. It leaves the left ventricle and arches posteriorly to the left side of the spinal column. This position is maintained as the aorta continues through the diaphragm to about the level of the navel. Here it divides into the right and left iliac arteries, which supply blood to the pelvis and legs (Figure 3-2).

Three major arteries branch off the aorta shortly after it leaves the heart. The first branch is the brachiocephalic artery. After traveling a short distance, it divides into the right common carotid (which carries blood to the brain, right eye) and right subclavian (which supplies blood to the right arm). Aortic branch number two is the left carotid. It carries blood to the brain and left eye. The third branch of the aorta is the left subclavian artery, which supplies blood to the left arm. As it descends in the body, the aorta gives off other branches to the lungs, esophagus, chest wall, diaphragm, kidneys, and intestines.

Veins

The superior vena cava returns blood to the heart from the upper half of the body. It is formed by the right and left brachiocephalic veins. These veins return blood from the right and left sides of the upper body respectively.

The right and left iliac veins, which carry blood from the legs and the pelvis, converge to form the inferior vena cava. The inferior vena cava returns blood from the lower half of the body to the heart.

Capillaries

Capillaries are very small blood vessels that join the arterial and venous systems. It is here that nutrients are delivered to the tissues, and blood takes up waste products from the tissues.

Blood

Blood is the tissue contained within blood vessels. The average person has between 4 and 6 liters of blood in his or her body. Plasma and cells are the two main parts of blood.

Plasma is mostly water (greater than 90%) and forms the liquid part of the blood. Other components of plasma include electrolytes (ie, sodium, potassium, calcium, and magnesium), glucose, fats, and proteins.

Cells form the solid component of blood. There are three types of blood cells: leukocytes (white blood cells), erythrocytes (red blood cells), and platelets.

Leukocytes form a major part of the body's defense mechanism against disease. When germs invade, leukocytes are mobilized to attack and destroy the intruders.

Erythrocytes produce the blood's red color. A molecule called hemoglobin, contained within the erythrocyte, transports oxygen from the lungs and releases it to the tissues. Carbon dioxide produced by the tissues is carried back to the lungs by erythrocytes, where it is exhaled into the environment.

Platelets help stop bleeding. When a break occurs in a blood vessel, the platelets congregate at that spot and plug up the hole.

Physiology

The muscle of the heart contracts on a regular basis (average is about 70 times per minute),

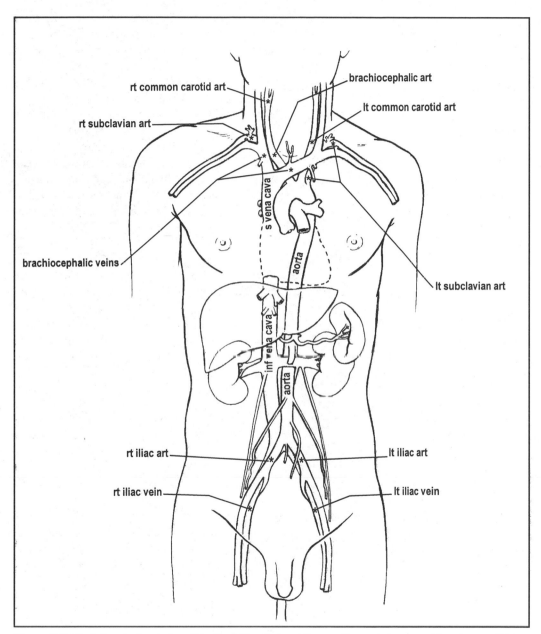

Figure 3-2. Peripheral circulation (Medical Illustration Library, General Anatomy Two image GA2-1039; Williams and Wilkins: 1994).

producing the heartbeat. With each contraction, blood surges down the arteries and can be felt as a pulse at the wrist, neck, and other places in the body.

Three things determine heart rate: the sympathetic nerves, parasympathetic nerves, and blood pressure.

Sympathetic nerves cause the heart to go faster. Things like fear and pain stimulate them. Parasympathetic nerves slow the heart rate. Pressure on the eyeball and vomiting slow the heart rate via the parasympathetic nerves. When blood pressure falls, the heart rate will increase. This is the body's way of returning the pressure back to normal. Raising the blood pressure, on the other hand, will cause the pulse to decrease.

Because it possesses the property of automaticity (the ability to initiate a heartbeat), the SA node originates the heartbeat. Under normal conditions, the SA node also determines how fast the heart contracts. The heartbeat begins as an electrical impulse. On leaving the SA node, it travels through atrial muscle fibers to the AV node. The AV node slows the impulse to allow maximal efficiency in heart muscle contraction. After exiting the AV node, the electricity travels down the Bundle of His, through the right and left bundle branches, ending in the muscles of the ventricles. The ventricular muscles then contract causing blood to flow to the lungs and rest of the body.

When pumping blood, the ventricles contract and relax. During contraction, the blood is squeezed into surrounding blood vessels. During relaxation, blood from the atria refills the ventricles in anticipation of the next contraction. The contraction is called systole, and the relaxation is called diastole.

Blood vessels are filled with blood at all times. Like water in the pipes of your house, the blood inside blood vessels is under pressure. When a vessel is violated (ie, a cut), the pressure within the vessel forces blood out through the hole, causing bleeding. Blood pressure is routinely measured as one of our vital signs. During systole, pressure in the vessel goes up, as the heart pumps blood out. This is called the systolic blood pressure. When the heart relaxes during diastole, pressure drops in the blood vessels. This is called the diastolic pressure. When blood pressure is recorded, the systolic pressure is written above the diastolic pressure. Systolic blood pressure will always be the higher of the two. The average normal blood pressure is 120/80.

Hemostasis means stopping the flow of blood. After an injury, this is very important because a very small injury would cause a person to bleed to death if hemostasis did not occur. Three things cause the body to stop bleeding after an injury: constriction of the blood vessel, platelets, and blood coagulation.

When a vessel is injured, the muscles making up the vessel wall contract. This makes the vessel smaller and restricts or stops blood flow. In addition, platelets move to the injured area and stick to it. As more and more platelets adhere to the site, a plug is formed. This also helps stop the flow of blood out of the vessel.

Blood clotting occurs when blood is changed from a liquid to a solid or semi-solid. The blood clot that results is formed by a complex reaction among several chemicals in the blood. The end product of the reaction is a protein called fibrin. Fibrin forms a meshwork at the site of injury that traps blood cells and other blood products. The resulting clot forms a dam, which helps prevent further bleeding.

Effects on the Eye

The cardiovascular system affects the eye in four ways: tissue support, infection control, hemostasis, and intraocular pressure regulation.

The tissues of the eye, such as the iris and retina, require oxygen and nutrients. If these are denied, the tissue stops functioning and eventually dies. Oxygen and nutrients are delivered to eye tissues by the cardiovascular system.

When infection invades the eye, cells and chemicals, which attack germs, are moved to the site of infection by the heart and blood vessels. These cells and chemicals control infection, helping to prevent ocular damage. This process usually causes inflammation, such as the redness seen with conjunctivitis.

Uncontrolled bleeding in the eye is a very serious problem that could lead to blindness. Platelets and clotting factors brought to the eye by the cardiovascular system help stop any bleeding that might occur. Thus, problems such as hyphema (bleeding into the anterior chamber) are usually limited and cause no permanent damage to the eye.

Pressure in the veins of the eye helps to produce intraocular pressure. Thus, large changes in the pressure of these veins can alter pressure inside the eye.

Chapter 4

The Respiratory System

OptT

OptA

KEY POINTS

- Oxygen is vital to the existence of cells.
- Carbon dioxide is the primary waste product of energy production.
- The respiratory system supplies oxygen to cells and expels carbon dioxide from the body.

Anatomy

The respiratory system has two divisions: the upper respiratory tract (Figure 4-1) and lower respiratory tract (Figure 4-2).

Upper Respiratory Tract

The nasal cavity is a hollow place in the skull directly above the mouth. It is separated from the mouth by the palate or "roof" of the mouth. The palate is easily felt by placing a finger in the uppermost portion of the mouth. Bone and cartilage make up the nasal septum, which divides the nasal cavity into two parts. Each part has a facial opening called a naris. Air first enters the respiratory system through the nares. Mucus and hair covering the inner surface of the nose trap dirt particles inhaled while breathing, preventing foreign material from getting into the lungs. The nose also adds heat and humidity to inhaled air, stopping the damage that drying would cause to the respiratory system.

Surrounding the nasal cavity are four pairs of air-filled spaces called sinuses. Voice quality during speaking or singing is partially determined by the sinuses. The maxillary sinuses are just below the eyes, the frontal sinuses are just above the eyes, the ethmoid sinuses are behind the frontal sinuses on either side of the nasal cavity, and the sphenoid sinuses are behind the nose just below the pituitary gland at the base of the brain. The sinuses are susceptible to infection during the cold and flu season. Symptoms include facial pain and a foul smelling nasal drainage.

The lateral walls of the nasal cavity have three bony protrusions called turbinates. They are named the superior, middle, and inferior turbinates. Openings beneath the middle turbinate connect to the frontal, ethmoid, and maxillary sinuses. The nasolacrimal duct empties tears under the inferior turbinate, and from here the tears go down the throat or out the nose. (Medications instilled into the eye follow the same path.)

The pharynx is the passageway between the nasal cavity and the larynx or voice box. Its purpose is to direct air into the trachea and carry food to the esophagus. The pharynx has three parts:
- the nasopharnyx begins where the nasal cavity ends, and is located above the back portion of the palate
- the oropharynx lies below the back portion of the palate behind the mouth. It is visible when looking into the mouth
- the laryngopharynx begins at the level of the larynx and ends at the esophagus

The oropharynx is shared by the respiratory and digestive systems as both food and air pass through it. A flap of tissue, the epiglottis, seals off the entrance to the larynx, thus denying food any access to the lower respiratory system. Commonly known as the Adam's apple, the larynx is responsible for the sound of the voice. The vocal cords are stretched across the inside of the larynx like the strings on a guitar. As air passes through the cords they vibrate, producing sound.

Lower Respiratory Tract

The trachea, commonly known as the windpipe, begins at the bottom of the larynx and forms the first part of the lower respiratory tract. A series of cartilage rings joined together by muscle and other tissues give shape and strength to the trachea, preventing it from collapsing during breathing or coughing. Behind the sternum (breastbone) in the center of the chest, the trachea divides into two directions. Each division is called a bronchus. One bronchus goes to the right lung and the other to the left lung. Once in the lung, the bronchi branch several more times, penetrating into increasingly smaller segments of the lung. Bronchioles are small extensions of the bronchi (less than 1 mm in diameter). They carry the air from the bronchi to the alveoli. Alveoli are sac-like structures at the end of the bronchioles that comprise the "business end" of the lungs.

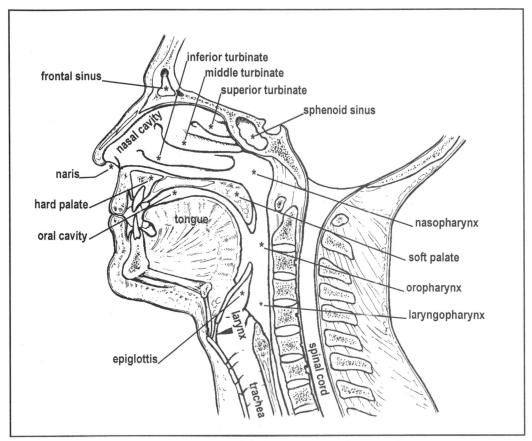

Figure 4-1. Upper respiratory tract (Medical Illustration Library, General Anatomy Two image GA2-4002; Williams and Wilkins: 1994).

Capillaries are stationed in close proximity to each alveolus. Because the walls of both capillaries and alveoli are thin, gasses move readily back and forth between them. It is here that oxygen moves into the blood from the alveoli, and carbon dioxide moves out of the blood into the alveoli.

Each lung is divided into segments called lobes. The right lung has three lobes—the upper lobe, middle lobe, and lower lobe. The left lung has two lobes, the upper lobe and the lower lobe. Each lobe is supplied with air by a branch of the bronchi. Both lungs, as well as the inside of the chest wall, are covered with a thin tissue called pleura. Pleurisy results when this tissue becomes inflamed, causing pain during breathing.

While not part of the respiratory system proper, the diaphragm and intercostal muscles play a critical role in its function. The diaphragm is a large muscle that separates the chest from the abdomen. It attaches to the lower ribs and vertebrae, and spans the entire inner circumference of the chest just below the lungs. The intercostal muscles fill the space between the ribs. They are attached to the ribs and move the ribs during breathing.

Physiology

Respiration is the process of taking oxygen into the body and transferring it to the blood stream for transport to cells. The respiratory system exists for this purpose. Ventilation and perfusion are two components of respiration.

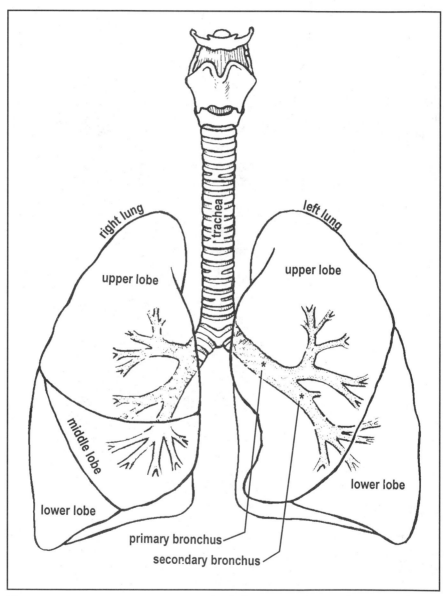

Figure 4-2. Lower respiratory tract (Medical Illustration Library, General Anatomy Two image GA2-4016; Williams and Wilkins: 1994).

Ventilation moves oxygen into the lungs and carbon dioxide out of the lungs. This is accomplished during the mechanical process called breathing. The respiratory control center in the brain sends out regular, subconscious electrical impulses that initiate breathing. It begins with the contraction of the diaphragm and intercostal muscles. As they contract, the chest and lungs expand. The expanding lungs suck in air from the environment (inhalation). Like a rubber band, the chest and lungs then spring back to their original shape, resulting in exhalation. This expels carbon dioxide transferred into the lungs from the bloodstream.

Breathing is regulated in two ways. Sensors in the lung and chest wall measure tension, speed of muscle contraction, movement during breathing, and other parameters. Based on these measurements, the body adjusts its breathing for greatest efficiency. Other sensors in the carotid artery, aorta and brain measure oxygen and carbon dioxide levels in the blood. When carbon dioxide levels rise, breathing is increased to get rid of it. When oxygen levels decrease, breathing increases to get more of it. The normal adult breathes about 12 times per minute. Breathing rate can be measured by counting the number of times the chest expands and contracts over a period of one minute.

Perfusion refers to blood flow in the lungs. Having oxygen in the lungs is of no value to the body unless it is delivered to the cells. Blood in capillaries that travel in close proximity to the alveoli receives oxygen and carries it to the cells of the body. Any interruption of blood flow to the lungs blocks oxygen transport to the cells, and with time, causes death.

Ventilation and perfusion must be balanced for respiration to be effective. If there is inadequate ventilation, there will be no oxygen available for the blood to transport to the cells. If there is inadequate perfusion, oxygen in the alveoli will remain there and not be transported to the cells.

Effects on the Eye

The respiratory system's effect on the eye is related to the supply of oxygen to and elimination of carbon dioxide from the tissues of the eye. Low levels of oxygen in the blood cause tissue malfunction and damage. Impaired contrast sensitivity, chronic pain, high or low intraocular pressure, glaucoma, and decreased night vision are a few of the eye problems that occur when the respiratory system does not supply enough oxygen to the eye. High levels of oxygen cause retinal damage in premature infants. Elevated carbon dioxide levels can cause mydriasis, increased intraocular pressure, and changes in blood flow to the eye.

Chapter 5

The Endocrine System

OptT

OptA

KEY POINTS

- Without the ability to adjust to a constantly changing internal and external environment, the body would soon die.

- Maintaining homeostasis in the face of these forces is a major function of the endocrine system.

- Controlling different actions and processes within the body allows the endocrine system to fill this role.

- The endocrine system frequently works in tandem with the nervous system.

Introduction

The body has two types of glands. Exocrine glands secrete their products through tube-shaped ducts. Salivary glands and sweat glands are two examples of exocrine glands.

In contrast, endocrine glands secrete their products directly into the blood, bypassing the need for ducts.

Each endocrine gland produces specific results in its target tissues. These effects are caused by chemicals called hormones. Each gland secretes unique hormones that cause the desired results. Because hormones have a wide range of powerful effects on the body, it is important that the quantities produced be closely regulated. The primary mechanism of hormone regulation is called negative feedback. Every hormone creates an effect in another part of the body. For example, insulin is the hormone secreted by the pancreas that causes the blood glucose level to drop. The effect of the hormone (the blood glucose level decreasing) turns off hormone production in its gland of origin (the pancreas stops producing insulin). As the insulin levels drop, its effect diminishes, and blood glucose levels begin to rise again. The pancreas responds by secreting more insulin. This negative feedback mechanism prevents the blood sugar from falling too low or going too high. In this manner, the quantity of hormone is adjusted to levels that are beneficial to the body. Other hormones in the body are controlled in a similar fashion.

Five different glands make up the endocrine system: pituitary, thyroid, parathyroid, pancreas, and adrenal glands.

Pituitary Gland

Like the control tower at an airport, the pituitary gland directs the actions of many other glands in the body. Because of this, it is known as the master gland. Located at the base of the brain, the pituitary gland is enclosed in a bony cavity known as the sella turcica (Figure 5-1).

The section of the brain immediately adjacent to the pituitary is the hypothalmus. It plays an important role in regulating the actions of the pituitary. The hypothalmus collects messages for the pituitary from other parts of the body. It then relays these instructions to the pituitary by chemicals known as releasing hormones. Releasing hormones cause the pituitary to release its different hormones. There are specific releasing hormones for each pituitary hormone.

An extension of the hypothalmus, called the infundibulum, connects it to the pituitary gland. The optic nerves cross near the pituitary gland, forming the optic chiasm. This relationship is important because tumors of the pituitary gland can put pressure on the optic nerves, causing changes in vision.

The pituitary gland has two parts—the posterior pituitary (neurohypophysis) and the anterior pituitary (adenohypophysis).

The posterior pituitary secretes hormones that are similar to chemicals in the nervous system. Vasopressin or antidiuretic hormone (ADH) causes the kidneys to conserve water. When the body doesn't take in enough fluid, the blood becomes more concentrated. In order to conserve water, the posterior pituitary secretes ADH. This signals the kidneys to stop getting rid of water. As a result, more water is retained in the body, and the blood concentration is restored to normal.

Oxytocin, another posterior pituitary hormone, has two actions. When an infant sucks his mother's breast, it causes a release of oxytocin from the posterior pituitary of the mother. Within a short time it reaches the cells of the breast, causing them to release milk to the nursing infant. For this reason, oxytocin is sometimes referred to as the milk letdown factor. In addition, oxytocin causes the uterus to contract and push the baby into the birth canal during childbirth.

The anterior pituitary secretes a number of different hormones:

1. Growth hormone exerts its primary effects during childhood and adolescence, stimulating

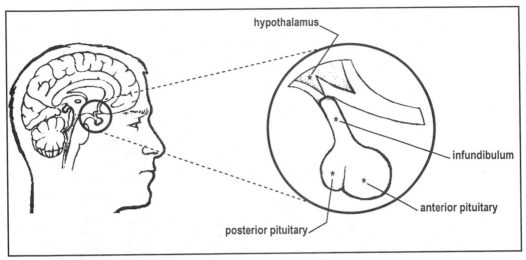

Figure 5-1. Pituitary gland (Medical Illustration Library, General Anatomy Two image GA2-7002; Williams and Wilkins: 1994).

the growth of bone and muscle. If not present in appropriate quantities, growth will not be normal.

2. Prolactin acts on the female breast during pregnancy. It is the primary hormone that causes the breast to secrete milk.
3. Thyroid stimulating hormone (TSH) stimulates the thyroid gland to produce the hormone thyroxine.
4. Follicle stimulating hormone (FSH) prompts the ovary and testicle to secrete the female hormone estrogen.
5. In response to luteinizing hormone (LH), the ovary and testicle release the male hormone testosterone.
6. Adrenocorticotropic hormone (ACTH) targets the adrenal gland, causing the release of multiple hormones.

Thyroid Gland

The thyroid gland is located in front of the trachea just below the larynx (Figure 5-2). It has two lobes connected by a narrow band of tissue called the isthmus. The shape of the gland is much like that of a butterfly. Thyroxine is the main hormone secreted by the thyroid gland, and its function is to control the body's rate of metabolism. For example, thyroxine helps determine the rate of oxygen usage by the body, causes the body temperature to go up, and increases the heart rate and force with which it contracts. Thyroid hormone also plays a critical role in the physical and mental development of infants. Its lack during infancy results in severe mental and physical impairment.

Parathyroid Glands

There are four parathyroid glands located on the posterior part of the thyroid gland. Parathormone (PTH) is the hormone secreted by the parathyroids. Its overall effect is to increase calcium levels in the blood. Two actions accomplish this: preventing excretion of calcium by the kidneys and removing calcium from the bones into the blood stream.

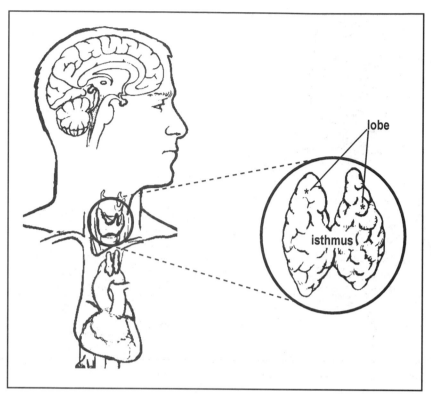

Figure 5-2. Thyroid gland (Medical Illustration Library, General Anatomy Two image GA2-7002; Williams and Wilkins: 1994).

Pancreas

The pancreas is located in the abdomen behind the stomach (Figure 5-3). It is both an exocrine and an endocrine gland. The exocrine part of the gland secretes digestive enzymes through a duct into the intestines. The endocrine part of the gland is called the islets of Langerhans. These are small clusters of several hundred cells scattered throughout the pancreas. Insulin and glucagon are the primary hormones secreted by the islet cells.

Insulin causes cells to draw glucose out of the blood, producing a drop in blood glucose levels. Glucagon stimulates cells to release glucose into the blood causing the level to increase. Working together, these two hormones help keep the blood glucose in a normal range.

Adrenal Glands

The adrenal glands are located in the abdomen on top of the kidneys (Figure 5-4). Each gland is made up of two parts—the medulla (which forms the center of the gland) and the cortex (which forms the outer part of the gland and surrounds the medulla).

The cortex secretes three primary hormones:

1. Aldosterone causes the kidneys to retain sodium and get rid of potassium. Retaining sodium helps maintain blood volume. High blood potassium levels interfere with heart function and can lead to cardiac arrest. Aldosterone prevents potassium levels from going too high.
2. Cortisol affects many different areas of the body. It helps regulate metabolism and supports the vascular system's ability to maintain blood pressure.

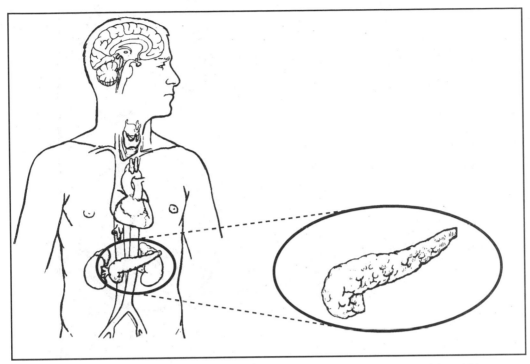

Figure 5-3. Pancreas (Medical Illustration Library, General Anatomy Two image GA2-7002; Williams and Wilkins: 1994).

3. Androgens are male sex hormones that affect sexual characteristics in both men and women.

The medulla secretes two very similar hormones—epinephrine (adrenaline) and norepinephrine. Both of these hormones prepare the body for action by increasing alertness, raising the blood pressure, and increasing the heart rate.

Effects on the Eye

The effects of the endocrine glands on the eye are due to specific disease states. These will be discussed in later chapters.

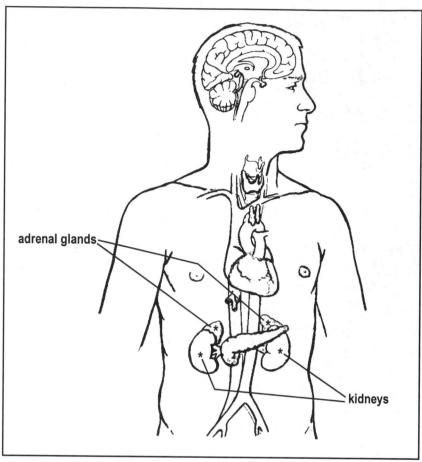

Figure 5-4. Adrenal glands (Medical Illustration Library, General Anatomy Two image GA2-7002; Williams and Wilkins: 1994).

Chapter 6

The Nervous System

OptT

OptA

KEY POINTS

- The nervous system directs and coordinates most of the body's activities.

- Directly or indirectly, the nervous system affects every part of the body.

- More than any other system, it gives the body a sense of "aliveness."

- Very short periods of time without necessary nutrients can cause permanent damage to the nervous system.

- The cells of the nervous system do not replace themselves.

Anatomy

The nervous system has two parts: the central nervous system and the peripheral nervous system.

Central Nervous System

The brain and spinal cord make up the central nervous system (Figure 6-1). When viewed together they look much like a round lollipop, the candy representing the brain, and the stick the spinal cord.

Brain

The brain is the largest and most complex component of the nervous system. It weighs approximately 1500 grams and is housed inside the skull, which provides protection for this most delicate of organs.

Four hollow spaces inside the brain are called ventricles. Ventricles help support the brain and act as conduits for the cerebrospinal fluid (see below). There are four ventricles—two lateral ventricles, the third ventricle, and the fourth ventricle.

Three layers of tissue cover the brain. These are the dura mater, arachnoid, and pia mater. The dura mater is the tough fibrous outermost covering. Its outer layer is adherent to the inner aspect of the skull. The optic nerve is covered by the dura. The arachnoid is a thin, membranous layer of connective tissue lying immediately beneath the dura. The innermost of the three layers is the pia mater, which adheres directly to the surface of the brain.

Between the arachnoid and pia mater is a water-like substance called the cerebrospinal fluid (CSF). It surrounds the entire brain and spinal cord. The CSF is produced by clumps of dilated capillaries inside the ventricles, called the choroid plexus. Once produced, the fluid travels through the ventricles, exits the brain, flows beneath the arachnoid, and finally is absorbed into the blood stream. A normal adult has approximately 130 cc of cerebrospinal fluid, which is replaced three to four times every 24 hours. The presence of CSF creates pressure inside the head (intracranial pressure). Blocking the circulation of the CSF causes the intracranial pressure to increase. If the pressure stays high for a number of days, it will cause elevation of the optic nerve head. This can be seen clinically on a funduscopic exam and is called papilledema.

The brain includes three major divisions: the brainstem, cerebellum, and cerebral cortex (Figure 6-2).

The brainstem is formed by the medulla oblongata, pons, midbrain, and diencephlon, and is responsible for many physiologic functions necessary for life (Figure 6-3). All of the cranial nerves, except the first and second (the cranial nerves are discussed later), originate from the brainstem.

The medulla oblongata is the lowest part of the brain and connects directly to the spinal cord. This area is shaped like a cylinder and is about 2.5 cm in length. The accessory, vestibulocochlear, glossopharyngeal, vagus, and hypoglossal nerves begin in the medulla.

Just in front of the medulla is a large, oblong section of brain called the pons. The pons, which means bridge, acts as a link between the medulla and other parts of the nervous system. The abducens, trigeminal, and facial nerves arise in the pons.

The next brainstem segment is called the midbrain. It controls eye motions produced by the oculomotor and trochlear cranial nerves. In addition, focusing the lens, pupillary size, and ocular convergence are regulated by this area.

The most forward section of the brainstem is the diencephon. It forms the gateway to the cerebrum. All signals entering and leaving the cerebrum pass through the diencephlon, thus exerting major control over brain performance. The optic nerves enter at the level of the diencephlon and

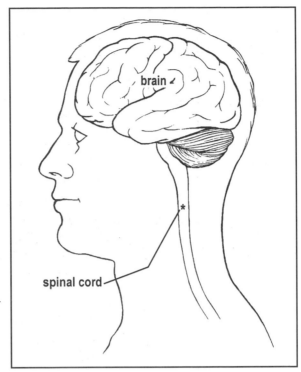

Figure 6-1. Central nervous system (Medical Illustration Library, General Anatomy Three image H301024; Williams and Wilkins: 1994).

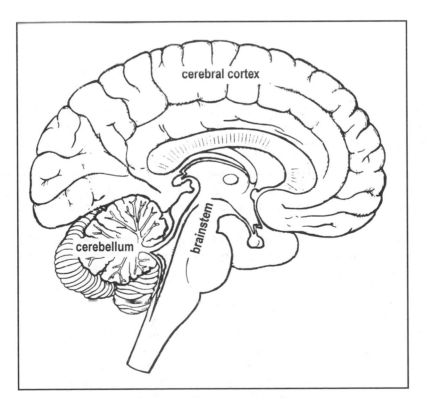

Figure 6-2. Three major divisions of the brain (sagittal section) (Mediclip, Human Anatomy Three image H301026; Williams and Wilkins).

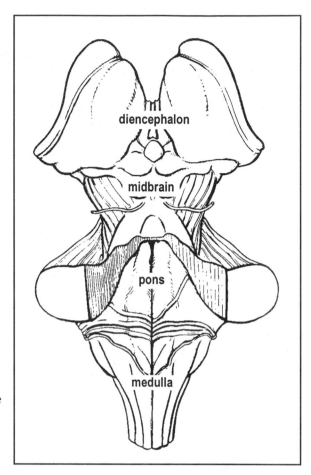

Figure 6-3.
Brainstem
(Mediclip,
Human Anato-
my Three image
H301016;
Williams and
Wilkins).

cross beneath it to form the optic chiasm. A major section of the diencephlon is the hypothalmus. It controls the pituitary gland, regulates body temperature, controls appetite, and produces physical expressions of emotions.

Located behind the brainstem is the second major area of the brain, the cerebellum. It synchronizes actions of muscle groups, producing smooth, coordinated motion. This includes muscles producing larger movements, such as sitting and standing, as well as those causing the finer movements of arms, legs, and hands. Dysfunction of the cerebellum produces erratic, disorganized motion of the body.

The third and largest part of the brain is the cerebrum, or the cerebral cortex (Figure 6-4). It forms the uppermost part of the brain. Many of the characteristics that make us uniquely human, such as speech, critical thinking, and personality, are produced in this area. The cerebrum is divided into right and left cerebral hemispheres. Each hemisphere is further divided into four lobes—frontal, parietal, occipital, and temporal.

The frontal lobe is the forward-most and largest part of the cerebral cortex. Signals from this area cause body movement to occur. In addition, personality, problem-solving ability, and reasoning are primarily the result of frontal lobe function.

The occipital lobe forms the posterior part of the cerebrum. It translates information from the retina into images that we can recognize. The right occipital cortex interprets information from the right half of each retina, and the left occipital cortex handles signals from the left half of each retina.

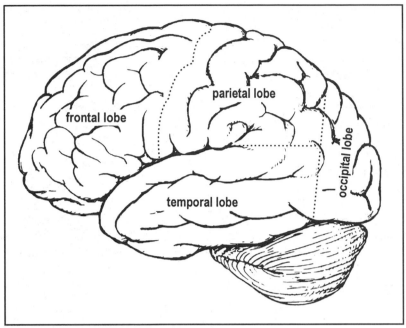

Figure 6-4. Cerebral cortex (Mediclip, Human Anatomy Three image H30100; Williams and Wilkins).

Sandwiched between the frontal and occipital lobes is the parietal lobe. Sensory information from many parts of the body is received and catalogued here.

The temporal lobe lies beneath the frontal and parietal lobes. It deals with sound perception and interpretation. Odor recognition also occurs in the temporal lobe.

Spinal Cord

The spinal cord is the second major part of the central nervous system. It is a slender, hose-like cylinder that begins at the medulla oblongata and extends 16 to 17 inches down the back. Surrounding the cord is the bony spinal canal formed by the vertebrae of the back, giving the spinal cord protection and stability. Signals traveling to and from the brain do so via the spinal cord. Peripheral nerves connect to the spinal cord through 31 pairs of spinal nerves. The spinal cord has four parts:

- the cervical cord (in the neck)
- the thoracic cord (running the length of the chest to just below the ribs)
- the lumbar cord (extending from just below the ribs to the level of the pelvic bone)

The spinal cord proper ends with the lumbar cord, but a large group of spinal nerves known as the cauda equina, extends further into the pelvis and is considered the fourth part of the spinal cord.

The Peripheral Nervous System

The peripheral nervous system is composed of nerves that travel to and from the brain and spinal cord. Those nerves that come from the brain are cranial nerves, while those from the spinal cord are spinal nerves. Both types of nerves branch many times in order to service the entire body. The central nervous system is linked with the rest of the body and the surrounding environment by the peripheral nervous system. There are two types of peripheral nerves. Motor nerves end in muscle and produce motion or other types of action. Sensory nerves transmit information from all parts of the body to the spinal cord and brain. They give us the ability to feel pain and touch, as well as differences in temperature and pressure.

The brain gives rise to 12 pairs of cranial nerves. They perform special functions primarily in the head and neck area. Each cranial nerve is assigned a number from 1 to 12. Following is a list of the cranial nerves and their actions:

I.   Olfactory—Carries information from the nose to the brain. It is responsible for the sense of smell.

II.   Optic—Carries information from the retina to the brain. It is a major factor in our ability to see.

III.   Oculomotor—Controls all extraocular muscles except the superior oblique and lateral rectus. It also innervates the superior levator palpebrae (which raises the upper eyelid), functions in pupillary dilation, and controls accommodation.

IV.   Trochlear—The smallest cranial nerve. Controls the superior oblique muscle.

V.   Trigeminal—The largest cranial nerve. It has three major branches:
- Ophthalmic: Controls sensation to the forehead, eyelids, nose, eyeball, conjunctiva, lacrimal gland, and inside of the nose and sinuses.
- Maxillary: Controls sensation to the lower eyelids, sides of the nose, upper lip, mouth, and sinuses.
- Mandibular—Controls sensation over the lower part of the face as well as to the teeth and gums, motor function to the chewing muscles.

VI.   Abducens—Controls function of the abducens muscle of the eye.

VII.   Facial—Controls function of facial expression muscles. It is responsible for taste on the anterior two-thirds of the tongue and sensation in the mouth and ear canal.

VIII.   Vestibulocochlear—Responsible for balance and hearing.

IX.   Glossopharyngeal—Controls taste from the posterior one-third of the tongue and sensation from the mouth and ear.

X.   Vagus—Innervates a number of areas from the neck to the abdomen. It provides sensation for the gastrointestinal tract, respiratory tract, and the heart. It also helps control heart rate and contractions of the gastrointestinal tract and bladder wall.

XI.   Accessory—Controls muscles of the shoulder, neck, pharynx, and larynx.

XII.   Hypoglossal—Controls the muscles of the tongue.

Physiology

The neuron is the primary cell of the nervous system (Figure 6-5). It has three parts: the body, dendrite, and axon. The body of the neuron processes and relays the information it receives. Dendrites are multiple tree-like projections from the neuron's body which receive information from other neurons. A single axon protrudes from the body of each neuron. It carries impulses away from the neuron to other neurons. Neurons are linked together to form pathways over which information, in the form of electrical current, is transmitted. These pathways form complex networks of interconnections that carry instructions to all parts of the body. The order of current flow through a pathway of the nervous system is dendrite, body of neuron, axon, dendrite (or body) of adjacent cell, axon of adjacent neuron, and so on. Parts of neurons don't actually touch one another when they transfer information. There is a small space called a synapse between the axon of one cell and the dendrite or body of the next. Information is transmitted across the synapse by chemicals called neurotransmitters.

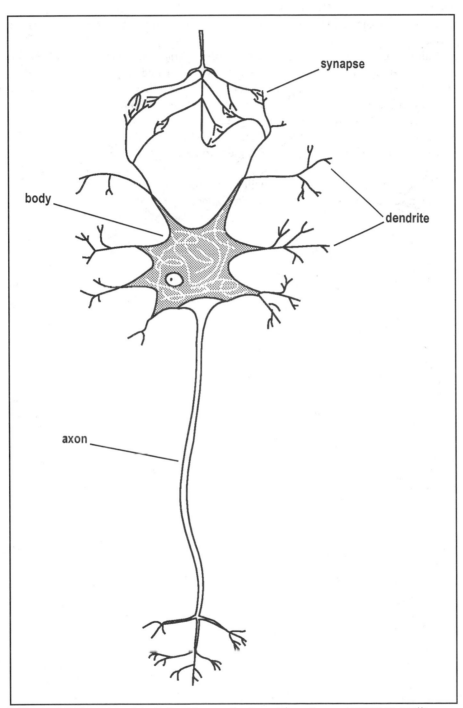

Figure 6-5. A neuron (Mediclip, Human Anatomy Three image H301040; Williams and Wilkins).

Effects on the Eye

Cranial nerves II through VII are all involved in normal eye function.

The optic nerve transmits visual images from the retina to the brain. Without it, vision would be impossible.

The oculomotor nerve causes muscle contraction in and around the eye. It innervates the superior rectus, which elevates the eye; the inferior rectus, which depresses the eye; the medial rectus, which directs the eye medially; the inferior oblique, which rotates the eye laterally; and the levator palpebrae superioris, which raises the upper eyelid. Additionally, it causes contraction of the sphincter muscle of the iris (constricting the pupil) and aids accommodation by contracting the ciliary muscle (allowing the lens to become thicker).

Medial rotation of the eye is produced by the trochlear nerve, which acts on the superior oblique. Lateral eye movement is produced by stimulation of the lateral rectus muscle by the abducens nerve. The trigeminal nerve supplies sensation to the eyeball and eyelids, while the facial nerve causes tear production by the lacrimal gland.

Chapter 7

Cardiovascular Disorders

KEY POINTS

- Ocular complications of endocarditis can include conjunctival and retinal hemorrhage, infection, and artery occlusion.

- Ocular complications of mitral valve prolapse can include occlusion of retinal blood vessels.

- Ocular complications of atherosclerosis and carotid artery disease can include retinal artery obstruction.

- Hypertension can cause narrowing, twisting, and fibrosis of retinal blood vessels.

- Retinal hemorrhage, papilledema, and cotton wool spots may also result from hypertension.

Endocarditis

Endocarditis is an infection of the lining or valves of the heart, commonly caused by bacteria such as strep or staph. In about half of the cases, the disease begins where there is damage to the heart lining or valve. Artificial heart valves also increase the risk of endocarditis. Both of these entities provide a place for bacteria to adhere to the heart and cause infection. The bacteria that cause endocarditis enter the blood stream after medical procedures, such as teeth cleaning or surgery, or by way of intravenous injections with dirty needles. In some patients the disease begins slowly with symptoms such as weakness, weight loss, fatigue, low grade fever, or loss of appetite. In others it begins more suddenly with chills, fever, and body aches.

Endocarditis alters blood flow through the heart causing a murmur (an abnormal noise heard while listening to the heart). The infection can also cause heart failure, blood clots to any part of the body, and stroke. Treatment is a multi-week regimen of appropriate antibiotics.

Conjunctival and retinal hemorrhages are ocular complications of endocarditis. The classic sign is a white-centered retinal hemorrhage called a Roth's spot. At times, infection in the heart will spread to the eye, causing vision-threatening infections. Blood clots and pieces of infected tissue can block arteries of the eye, depriving it of needed oxygen.

Mitral Valve Prolapse

When the left ventricle contracts, the mitral valve normally closes, preventing blood from returning to the atrium. In mitral valve prolapse (MVP), part of the valve stretches (prolapses) back into the atrium allowing some blood to return to the atrium. The blood leaking back into the atrium produces a heart murmur, which actually helps diagnose the disorder. An irregular heartbeat and rarely sudden death are associated with mitral valve prolapse. Patients with MVP are also at greater risk for developing endocarditis. Many people with this disease have abnormal platelet function. Normal platelets clump together and plug holes in blood vessels to stop bleeding. In mitral valve prolapse, the platelets are overactive and may cluster together even when the blood vessels are intact. These masses of platelets can travel to other places in the body, block blood vessels, and cause damage to organs. Approximately 5% of the population has mitral valve prolapse, and to date its cause is unknown. An echocardiogram (ultrasound of the heart) allows doctors to see the valve prolapsing back into the atrium and diagnose the disorder.

The ocular effects of mitral valve prolapse are due to platelet dysfunction. When abnormal clumps of platelets form, they can migrate to the eye, blocking blood vessels and denying needed oxygen and nutrients. This can cause impairment or loss of vision.

Atherosclerosis

Atherosclerosis refers to the build-up of fat in the arteries. This primarily affects large arteries, but can be seen in almost any artery of the body. The fatty deposits can block vessels, weaken the vessel wall (causing rupture and damage to adjacent organs), or form blood clots that can migrate to other areas of the body and cause damage. High blood cholesterol levels, smoking, and high blood pressure are major causes of atherosclerosis.

The symptoms and diseases caused by atherosclerosis are related to the arteries it affects. When the coronary arteries of the heart are involved, chest pain and heart attacks result. Strokes can occur when arteries of the brain are affected. Blockage of leg arteries causes leg pain and can necessitate amputation.

Effects of atherosclerosis on the eye are due to blockage of ocular arteries, causing partial or complete loss of vision. Either a build-up of fatty material obstructs the artery or pieces of fat or clotted blood travel to the eye and block an artery. These mechanisms are a frequent cause of central retinal artery occlusion.

Carotid Artery Disease

In the front part of the neck on either side of the trachea are two medium-sized arteries known as the carotid arteries. They are the main source of blood supply to the brain. By way of the internal carotids (branch arteries of the carotids), they also provide the primary blood supply to the eyes. The carotid arteries cause problems when they are restricted or blocked, usually by atherosclerotic plaques. When this occurs, oxygen supplies to the brain are restricted. Consequently, brain tissue dies (stroke), or a silent, slow, diffuse brain damage known as cerebral atrophy occurs.

Ocular damage results when pieces of plaque break off, migrate to the eye, and interrupt its blood supply. If the central retinal artery is blocked, there will be sudden, painless loss of vision. Permanent visual loss results if circulation is not restored within 100 minutes. Temporary blockage of eye arteries causes a few minutes of visual loss, known as amaurosis fugax.

Hypertension

Hypertension is a disease that elevates blood pressure and damages organs. Blood pressure is considered high when it is greater than 140/90. Damage occurs when it remains high over a protracted period of time or becomes very high very quickly. The organs most commonly damaged are the heart, brain, and kidneys. Most patients with this disease have no symptoms. Other patients develop headaches, dizziness, ringing in the ears, or nose bleeds. Malignant hypertension is a severe form of high blood pressure that is life-threatening. In these patients, the pressure rises very quickly and stays above 120 diastolic. Additionally, there is evidence of brain, heart, or kidney damage.

Ninety percent of hypertension has no known cause. The remaining 10% is due to kidney, adrenal, or other diseases. Untreated, high blood pressure can cause heart failure, heart attack, stroke, kidney failure, and even death. It is estimated that 15 million Americans have hypertension.

Retinal blood vessels are the primary ocular target of hypertension. The vessels narrow and become either straightened or twisted in appearance. The normal tissue in their walls is replaced by fibrous tissue, causing a copper or silver wire appearance on funduscopic exam. Retinal veins are compressed by the arteries that cross over them, giving them the appearance of being squeezed in or cut (AV nicking). Hemorrhage into the retina is typical. Some areas of the retina are completely cut off from their blood supply producing blurred, grayish white areas known as cotton wool patches. Particularly in malignant hypertension, the optic disc can swell (papilledema).

Chapter 8

Endocrine Disorders

| KEY POINTS |

- Diabetics have a higher incidence of glaucoma and cataracts than the general population.

- The ocular effects of diabetes can include leaking and rupture of retinal blood vessels, neovascularization, retinal detachment, and macular edema.

- Graves' disease, the leading cause of hyperthyroidism, can cause inflammation and swelling of the extraocular muscles, corneal exposure, and compression of the optic nerve.

- Ocular changes that can be associated with hypothyroidism include partial loss of brows and lashes, swelling, keratoconus, cataracts, and optic atrophy.

- Tumor of the pituitary gland may cause visual field loss, optic atrophy, and nerve palsy.

Diabetes

As discussed in Chapter 5, insulin is secreted by beta cells in the islet of Langerhans of the pancreas. The role of insulin is to regulate blood glucose levels. When the pancreas does not secrete enough insulin or when the insulin secreted is not effective, the blood glucose will be high. The resulting disease is called diabetes mellitus. Three classic symptoms of diabetes are polyuria (increased frequency of urination), polydipsia (increased thirst), and polyphagia (increased appetite). The diagnosis is made by finding high glucose levels in the blood.

There are two types of diabetes: type 1 (juvenile or insulin dependent diabetes), and type 2 (adult onset or non-insulin dependent diabetes). Type 1 diabetes usually begins before age 35 and comprises 10% of all diabetes. In this type of diabetes, pancreatic beta cells are destroyed causing very low blood insulin levels. Consequently, not enough insulin is present to keep blood glucose levels normal. These patients require insulin injections in order to survive. Causes of type 1 diabetes include genetic inheritance, viral infections of the pancreas, and destruction of the beta cells by the body's immune system.

Type 2 diabetes usually begins after age 35. While insulin levels are normal or high, the body does not respond properly and blood glucose levels elevate. Eventually the islet cells wear out and levels of insulin drop, making control of blood glucose even more difficult. Genetic inheritance, obesity, poor diet, lack of exercise, and stress have been implicated as causes for type 2 diabetes. Treatment for type 2 diabetes includes diet, exercise, and oral medications that lower blood glucose levels.

Diabetics have a higher incidence of glaucoma and cataracts than the general population. However, the most significant eye damage caused by diabetes involves the retina. Diabetic retinopathy is the second leading cause of permanent blindness and includes several changes to the eye.

In diabetics, small sac-like bulges occur in the walls of retinal blood vessels. These microaneurysms leak fluid and are prone to rupture, releasing blood into the retina. The fluid released by these and other leaky blood vessels cause retinal swelling. If swelling involves the macula, loss of visual acuity will result. Macular edema is the leading cause of blindness in diabetics. In patients with diabetic retinopathy, many small blood vessels of the retina become blocked. This denies the retina the oxygen it needs. Partially in response to this lack of oxygen, new, abnormal blood vessels form (neovascularization). These fragile vessels bleed into the vitreous, impairing vision. With time, the vessels start to shrink. As they do, retinal detachments can occur. The treatment for diabetic retinopathy is destruction of the new blood vessels using laser therapy.

Hyperthyroidism

Hyperthyroidism is caused by an overactive thyroid gland. Overactivity causes the gland to secrete high levels of thyroid hormone. Graves' disease is the most frequent cause of hyperthyroidism. It is characterized by an overactive and swollen thyroid gland (goiter). High thyroid hormone levels put the body's metabolism into overdrive causing anxiety, nervousness, and sometimes tremor. Heart rate increases and abnormal rhythms may occur. Patients are unable to tolerate heat, have increased appetites, and weight loss. There are three treatments for hyperthyroidism—drugs that block the gland's ability to produce or release thyroid hormone, radioactive iodine that destroys the gland's ability to produce thyroid hormone, and surgical removal of the thyroid gland.

Most of the ocular changes of Graves' disease are due to inflammation and swelling of the extraocular muscles. The muscle swelling pushes the eyeball forward, causing exophthalmus. This gives the patient the appearance of being startled or frightened. Over time the upper lid retracts, further exposing the eye. Consequently the cornea dries out, causing corneal abrasions and ulcers. This, along with compression of the optic nerve by swollen muscles, can result in loss of vision.

Hypothyroidism

Hypothyroidism is caused by an underactive thyroid gland. Low thyroid hormone levels result, causing the body's metabolic rate to slow down. Symptoms include general fatigue, weakness and lack of energy, intolerance to cold temperatures, weight gain, hair loss, dry skin, and enlarged tongue. Children born with hypothyroidism will have poor mental and physical development if not treated soon after birth. Taking thyroid hormone in pill form will reverse the effects of hypothyroidism.

Ocular changes caused by hypothyroidism include loss of the outer part of eyebrows and eyelashes; swelling of the conjunctival, corneal, and periorbital areas; keratoconus; cataracts; and optic atrophy.

Pituitary Adenoma

Pituitary adenoma is a tumor of the pituitary gland. It is the most common pituitary gland disorder and makes up 10% to 15% of all intracranial neoplasms. At autopsy, 25% of the adult population has pituitary adenomas. These tumors cause problems in one of two ways—either they change the amount of hormone the pituitary secretes or their size damages surrounding structures.

Adrenocorticotrophic hormone (ACTH), prolactin, and growth hormone are the most common hormones secreted by pituitary adenomas. The resulting high levels of these chemicals cause disorders such as Cushing's syndrome, acromegaly, and infertility. Prolactin-secreting adenomas are the most common type of these tumors.

Visual field loss and headaches are the most frequent presenting complaints of patients with large adenomas. These tumors can damage adjacent normal pituitary tissue causing hypopituitarism. If the adenoma extends outside the sella turcica, it can compress the optic chiasm or other adjacent structures. The typical physical finding with optic nerve involvement is bitemporal hemianopsia. If nerve compression is not relieved, optic atrophy and permanent visual loss may occur. Lateral spread of the tumor can cause III, IV, or VI nerve palsy. These patients complain of diplopia but usually have no visual field defects.

Pituitary apoplexy is caused by sudden hemorrhage into an adenoma. Symptoms include headache, confusion, vomiting, fever, loss of consciousness, decreased vision, and extraocular muscle paresis. The bleeding destroys pituitary tissue and creates a life-threatening problem that requires urgent surgery.

A computed tomography (CT) or magnetic resonance imaging (MRI) scan of the sella turcica and pituitary gland is used to diagnose a pituitary adenoma.

The drugs octreotide and bromocriptine are used to block hormonal effects and decrease the size of certain types of pituitary adenomas. When these drugs are not effective, surgical removal of the tumor is indicated. Postoperative radiation can help prevent recurrence when the tumor cannot be completely removed by surgery.

Small tumors that secrete no hormones usually require no treatment. Periodic MRI or CT scans are performed to monitor tumor size.

Chapter 9

Infectious Disease

OphA

KEY POINTS

- Acquired immunodeficiency syndrome (AIDS) damages retinal blood vessels, causing swelling and cotton wool patches.

- Herpes simplex type 1 is one of the most frequent causes of blindness due to corneal disease.

- Shingles (Varicella zoster) can cause lesions on the cornea and lids, as well as inflammation of the conjunctiva, sclera, and uvea.

- Ocular involvement with tuberculosis is very rare, but tubercles can occur in any part of the eye except the lens.

- The primary ocular complication of toxoplasmosis is chorioretinitis.

AIDS

AIDS is the abbreviation for acquired immunodeficiency syndrome. It is caused by the human immunodeficiency virus (HIV). As is suggested by its name, the HIV virus attacks the body's immune system, impairing its ability to combat disease. Thus, AIDS is characterized by the appearance of frequent, and many times rare, forms of infections and cancer. AIDS evolves very slowly. In fact, 50% of patients do not develop AIDS until 10 years after they are infected with HIV. In the majority of cases, infection with the HIV virus occurs by sexual contact or transmission of blood products (via blood transfusions or intravenous drug abuse). Ten to 40% of pregnant women with AIDS may also transmit the disease to their unborn child. At present there is no cure for AIDS, though several drugs can lessen the severity of the disease and possibly prolong life. Death is usually caused by infections or cancers that overwhelm the body's compromised immune system.

AIDS damages the blood vessels of the retina. Retinal blood flow is thus compromised, causing swelling and the appearance of cotton wool patches. This is the most common eye change seen in patients with AIDS. As with the rest of the immunocompromised body, the eye is more susceptible to infection. One of the most common eye infections in patients with AIDS is cytomegalovirus (CMV). This virus attacks and destroys the retina (see next section). Kaposi's sarcoma is a form of cancer that is frequently seen in AIDS patients. In 18% of patients, this cancer affects the eyelids, conjunctiva, or orbit. When present on the conjunctiva, it appears as a bright red diffuse lesion that may be mistaken for a subconjunctival hemorrhage. While the HIV virus can be found in tears of infected patients, there is no evidence to date that AIDS can be transmitted through tears.

Cytomegalovirus

Exposure to CMV is widespread, occurring in 80% of all adults at some point in their lives. Though most have no symptoms, low-grade fever and malaise are common when symptoms do occur. Its presentation is very similar to infectious mononucleosis. Most infections are minor and cause no long-term disability. In two instances, though, CMV can produce serious illness. Women infected during pregnancy can transmit the infection to their unborn baby. This may cause serious birth defects like mental retardation, seizures, and hearing loss. People with defective immune systems, such as AIDS patients, are also at risk for serious disease. In these patients, CMV can infect the eye, gastrointestinal tract, nervous system, or lungs. CMV is the most common cause of life-threatening viral infection in patients with AIDS.

Cytomegalovirus has little effect on the eye when the immune system is normal. However, when the immune system is damaged, as in AIDS, ocular CMV infections are common. CMV causes a diffuse retinitis characterized by swelling, bleeding, destruction of tissue, and detachment of the retina. Varying degrees of visual loss (including blindness) result. Twenty to 40% of all patients with AIDS will have an ocular CMV infection at some point in the course of their illness. The antiviral drug ganciclovir is used to treat CMV retinitis.

Epstein-Barr Virus

The Epstein-Barr (EB) virus causes infectious mononucleosis. Most cases of infectious mononucleosis occur in teenagers and young adults. This illness begins 30 to 40 days after exposure to the virus and is characterized by fatigue, malaise, muscle aches, fever, and sore throat. Lymph glands in the neck are swollen, and in some instances, the spleen and liver also enlarge.

The tonsils increase in size and are covered with heavy white exudates. Patients are usually symptomatic for up to 1 month. There is no effective treatment for infectious mononucleosis other than relief of symptoms.

Periorbital and eyelid edema are common in patients with infectious mononucleosis. While the conjunctiva is the most frequent site infected by the Epstein-Barr virus, it can also cause disease in the iris, sclera, or cornea. Optic neuritis and papilledema have also resulted from EB virus infection.

Herpes Simplex

There are two types of Herpes simplex virus (HSV). Type 1 HSV usually infects the mouth and face, while type 2 infects the genital area. Symptoms of herpes simplex infection begin 3 to 12 days after exposure and initially consist of local tenderness, fever, malaise, and loss of appetite. Blisters appear after 24 to 48 hours and subsequently rupture, leaving the painful ulcers that characterize the infection. Genital infections may be accompanied by penile or vaginal discharge. The ulcers heal over a 1- to 3-week period. After symptoms resolve, the virus takes up residence in local sensory nerves. From here, HSV can cause infection at any time without re-exposure. Treatment for genital herpes is the antiviral drug acyclovir. Treatment for oral herpes is symptomatic.

HSV causes more than 500,000 cases of corneal infections each year. It is one of the most frequent causes of blindness due to corneal disease. Symptoms of ocular involvement include foreign body sensation, irritation, tearing, and photophobia. Corneal ulceration is the primary physical finding. The classic ulcer looks like a branching tree (dendrite) when stained with fluoroscein. Healing usually occurs in 2 weeks with the use of antiviral drops such as vidarabine and acyclovir. HSV infection frequently leaves the cornea scarred or cloudy and the vision impaired.

Influenza

Influenza is a viral infection that frequently occurs in epidemics. The epidemics can last 6 weeks and may affect up to 20% of a given community. Children have the highest rate of infection. The disease is spread from person to person via coughing, sneezing, or other close contact. Symptoms include fever, chills, loss of appetite, muscle aches, headache, fatigue, dry cough, nasal discharge, and sore throat. Fever usually lasts 1 to 5 days. Cough may persist for 2 weeks after other symptoms resolve. The treatment for influenza is primarily symptomatic. However, certain types of influenza can be treated with antiviral drugs such as amantadine and rimantadine. Influenza vaccinations are available, but their effectiveness is variable. They are recommended for people at high risk for influenza or its complications (ie, healthcare workers, the elderly, etc).

Conjunctivitis may occur in the early stages of influenza. It may be accompanied by periorbital swelling or subconjunctival hemorrhage and usually lasts 4 to 5 days. Dacryoadenitis (infection of the lacrimal gland) also occurs with some frequency in the later stages of influenza.

Varicella Zoster

This virus causes two diseases: chickenpox and shingles. Chickenpox is primarily a disease of childhood, occurring most commonly in children 5 to 10 years of age. Most infections appear in the winter and spring. The disease begins 11 to 22 days after exposure to the Varicella virus. Its characteristic feature is a pruritic (itching) rash that begins on the face, neck, or upper trunk and spreads to the rest of the body. Lesions may also involve the mucous membranes of the mouth. The appearance of the rash goes through four stages—initially small firm sores, then blisters with clear fluid, then blisters with cloudy fluid, and finally ruptured blisters, which crust over. Fever, headache, muscle aches, and fatigue usually accompany the rash. Chickenpox is contagious from the day preceding rash until all lesions are crusted over (usually a total of 7 days). Most episodes of chickenpox are resolved in 7 to 10 days. Treatment is symptomatic, though in severe cases acyclovir can be used to lessen the intensity and duration of the disease. Chickenpox may cause conjunctivitis, which is the most common ocular involvement. Corneal infection may also occur but usually causes no permanent scarring.

After an episode of chickenpox, the Varicella virus can live for many years in sensory nerves of the body without causing symptoms. Reactivation of the virus can occur at any time, however, causing a typical chickenpox rash along the course of the nerve that the virus inhabits. This disease is called shingles or herpes zoster. Shingles usually begins with a burning pain along the course of the infected nerve, which may last for several days. In the absence of the typical rash, this can be mistaken for other diseases. The rash then appears, affecting only the skin over the involved nerve on one side of the body. Pain is frequently very severe. Nerves of the chest wall are most commonly infected followed by scalp, neck, and lower back. The pain and rash resolve in 3 to 4 weeks. Acyclovir can be used to lessen the severity of the infection and help prevent post-infection complications.

Shingles affects the eye when the Varicella virus inhabits the ophthalmic division of the trigeminal nerve. On reactivation, the virus causes the typical rash on the forehead, eyelids, and nose on one side of the face. About 75% of these patients will have eyeball involvement as well. If the tip of the nose is involved (it is innervated by the nasociliary branch of the ophthalmic nerve), there is a very high likelihood of corneal involvement. Lid lesions may result in damage and scarring that require oculoplastic surgery. Dysfunction of the extraocular muscles can occur due to involvement of the III, IV, and VI cranial nerves. Inflammation of the sclera and conjunctiva is common. Ulceration and opacification of the cornea may compromise vision. Uveitis is also a frequent finding. Treatment with acyclovir is effective in preventing many of the ocular complications of this disease.

Measles

Measles is a viral disease usually occurring in the winter and spring. Previously it infected primarily the 5 to 9 age group, but since the advent of a measles vaccine, young adults and others who have not been immunized are most often infected. It takes 7 to 10 days from the time of exposure for the disease to appear. Cough, runny nose, conjunctivitis, headache, and high fever last for 3 days. As these symptoms progress, small white spots (Koplik spots) appear inside the mouth on the cheeks. A red, irregular rash arises when fever is at its highest (usually about 14 days after exposure). It begins behind the ears and on the forehead, spreading from there over the face and rest of the body. After 3 or 4 days the rash begins to fade, usually resolving in 1 week. Treatment for measles is symptomatic. The measles vaccine, developed in 1963, has been effective in reducing the occurrence of this disease.

The majority of patients with measles develop conjunctivitis and watery discharge a few days before the rash appears. Subconjunctival hemorrhage may occur as well. Superficial keratitis is also common but resolves rapidly and causes no permanent scarring. No treatment is required for any of these problems.

Chlamydia

With 3 million cases appearing annually, chlamydia is the most common sexually transmitted infection in the United States. It is caused by the organism *Chlamydia trachomatis*. Symptoms begin 1 to 5 weeks after sexual contact with an infected partner. In men, it causes urethritis with symptoms such as pain on urination, white or clear penile discharge, and occasionally testicular or low abdominal pain. Chlamydia is also a frequent cause of epididymitis in men under 35. Sites of infection in women include the cervix, fallopian tubes, and urethra. When the fallopian tubes are involved, chronic pelvic pain, infertility, and ectopic pregnancy (pregnancy occurring outside of the uterus) can result. Many infected females are without symptoms, increasing the spread of the disease. When symptoms do occur, they include yellow vaginal discharge, pain, and frequency of urination, and when the fallopian tubes are involved, low abdominal pain can occur. During birth, babies of infected mothers have a 60% to 70% risk of contracting chlamydial infections such as pneumonia and conjunctivitis. Chlamydia can be successfully treated with tetracycline and other antibiotics.

In the United States, conjunctivitis due to chlamydia usually occurs in young sexually active adults who have been exposed to infected genital secretions. As mentioned above, infants born to infected mothers may also develop conjunctival infections.

From a global perspective, trachoma is the most significant ocular problem caused by chlamydia, affecting 600 million people worldwide. It rarely occurs in the United States, but is common in developing third world countries where there is poor sanitation and contaminated drinking water. Trachoma is a chronic chlamydial infection of the cornea and conjunctiva. Conjunctival infection causes scarring, which results in trichiasis and entropion. In response to the infection, blood vessels may develop in the cornea, obscuring vision. These entities further damage the cornea, ultimately resulting in blindness. Antibiotic treatment will cure trachoma, but the damage caused by the chlamydial infection is permanent.

Syphilis

Syphilis is a sexually transmitted disease caused by the organism *Treponema pallidum*. It occurs in three stages—primary, secondary, and tertiary syphilis.

Primary syphilis begins 2 to 6 weeks after exposure. It usually presents as a single, painless ulcer (chancre) at the site of sexual contact and lasts 1 to 6 weeks. Lymph nodes in the groin area may be enlarged as well. If no treatment is given, secondary syphilis begins 2 to 12 weeks later. Initially there are general symptoms such as muscle aches and sore throat, followed by widespread enlargement of lymph nodes. Subsequently a raised, non-itching rash appears and spreads over the entire body. Involvement of the palms of the hands, soles of the feet, and mucous membranes of the mouth and genital area are distinctive features of the rash. Many other areas of the body can be infected as well, including the liver, kidneys, eye, bone, stomach, and brain. A latent period of months to years precedes the development of tertiary syphilis. One third of untreated patients with secondary syphilis will develop tertiary syphilis. This stage causes damage to the brain, bones, skin, and aorta, and can be fatal. Syphilis can be transmitted from an infected woman to her unborn child. Primary and secondary syphilis can be cured with one shot of benzathine penicillin. Tertiary syphilis requires extended treatment with penicillin.

A chancre may appear on the conjunctiva or eyelids during primary syphilis. Other ocular effects occur during the secondary and tertiary stages. Many parts of the eye can be affected by this disease, including the lids, conjunctiva, lacrimal system, orbit, cornea, sclera, lens, iris, vitreous, retina, pupils, and optic nerve. When syphilis infects the brain, dysfunction of the oculomotor, trochlear, and abducens nerves may occur, causing extraocular muscle weakness. Optic nerve involvement causes swelling of the optic disc and optic atrophy, resulting in partial or complete visual loss. The classic finding in tertiary syphilis is the Argyll-Robertson pupil. Normal pupils are round, regular, and constrict in response to light and near visual effort. The Argyll-Robertson pupil, however, is small and irregular, and has little or no reaction to light. On near effort, though, it does constrict.

Tuberculosis

Tuberculosis is caused by the organism *Mycobacterium tuberculosis*. In recent years, tuberculosis has become a disease of the elderly, non-white, foreign born, and of patients with HIV infection. It is spread from person to person by infected secretions sent airborne by coughing and sneezing. Once in the body, the organism reproduces for 2 to 3 weeks and then spreads via the lymph system to all parts of the body. Symptoms rarely appear during this time and no further growth or spread of the bacteria occurs. After lying dormant for months to years, it may reactivate and cause symptomatic disease.

Tuberculosis most commonly presents as a lung infection such as pneumonia or an abscess. Symptoms such as night sweats, loss of appetite, fever, cough, shortness of breath, and weight loss accompany the infection. Many other sites in the body can become infected including the lymph nodes, liver, bones, gastrointestinal tract, urinary tract, eye, and meninges of the brain. Exposure to tuberculosis is tested by the purified protein derivative (PPD) skin test. This test is performed by injecting a small amount of protein from the tuberculosis bacteria under the skin of the forearm. Swelling will occur at the injection site if the patient has been exposed to the disease. Tuberculosis is treated with the medications isoniazid, rifampin, and pyrazinamide, which are usually taken for 6 months.

Ocular involvement with tuberculosis is rare, occurring in 1% to 2% of cases. The only part of the eye that isn't affected by the disease is the lens. The typical lesion of tuberculosis (the tubercle) can be found in any part of the eye, but is most commonly seen in the choroid.

Lyme Disease

Lyme disease was first described in 1975 in Old Lyme, Connecticut (hence the name). The causative organism, *Borrelia burgdorfen*, is carried by certain types of ticks and is transmitted when an infected tick bites a human. Lyme disease usually occurs in the summer, and one third of cases occur in children and teenagers. Symptoms begin 3 to 32 days after exposure and include fever, fatigue, muscle and joint pain, and swollen lymph glands. A red, raised, centrally clearing, expanding rash appears 1 to 8 weeks after the tick bite and is a distinctive feature of the disease. If not treated, arthritis, myocarditis (inflammation of muscle of heart), and abnormal cranial nerve function can result. Treatment with antibiotics such as amoxicillin or doxycycline is curative.

Relatively little is known about the effects of Lyme on the eye. In some studies, up to 11% of patients have conjunctivitis. Periorbital edema is occasionally seen. Corneal infiltrates, uveitis, and endophthalmitis have all been described in patients with Lyme disease.

Toxoplasmosis

Toxoplasma gondii is a parasite found primarily in cats and is the entity responsible for toxoplasmosis. The organism reproduces in cat's intestines and enters the soil from the feces. From here other animals (including cattle, pigs, and sheep) take it up. Humans acquire *Toxoplasma* in three ways: ingestion of infected, improperly cooked meat; contact with and ingestion of cat feces (ie, contamination of hands while cleaning a cat litter box); and transmission from an infected mother to her unborn baby. Infection in people with normal immune systems usually causes no symptoms. When symptoms do occur, they are similar to infectious mononucleosis with fever, malaise, sore throat, rash, swollen lymph nodes, and enlarged liver and spleen. Congenital infections cause chorioretinitis, mental retardation, and intracranial calcifications. Most infections occur in people with defective immune systems, such as AIDS or cancer patients. Severe brain, muscle, eye, and lung infections are common. Toxoplasmosis can be successfully treated with the medications sulfadiazine and pyrimethamine.

The majority of ocular toxoplasmosis results from activation of toxoplasma cysts planted in the retina during a congenital infection. Rarely does it result from an infection acquired later in life. Chorioretinitis is the primary ocular complication of toxoplasmosis. Infection begins with rupture of the toxoplasma cysts, producing retinal inflammation and invasion of retinal cells by the toxoplasma organism. The parasites multiply until the cells rupture and die. Depending on the number of cells involved and their location, visual acuity can be threatened. Other ocular complications include papillitis, papilledema, and vitritis.

Chapter 10

Connective Tissue Disease

KEY POINTS

- Scleritis is common in patients with serum lupus erythematosis.

- Multiple sclerosis is a common cause of optic neuritis.

- The most common ocular complication of rheumatoid arthritis is keratoconjunctivitis sicca.

- The most severe ocular complication of temporal arteritis is occlusion of the arteries supplying the optic nerve.

Serum Lupus Erythematosus

Serum lupus erythematosis (SLE) is an autoimmune disease, meaning that the immune system, which normally attacks foreign substances, attacks normal tissue. In SLE, the body's immune system attacks and damages connective tissue. Because connective tissue is found in most parts of the body, this illness involves many different systems. SLE occurs nine times more often in women than men, primarily affecting women of child bearing age. Black females contract SLE three times more often than white females. The most common symptoms of the illness include fever, weight loss, fatigue, arthritis, sensitivity to light, and a butterfly-shaped rash on the face. Tissues most often involved include the brain, kidney, lung, muscle, heart, joints, and blood. SLE may present in any one or several of these areas. The course of the disease varies from patient to patient, but exacerbations and remissions are usual. Sunlight, situational stress, infection, and some drugs (ie, procainamide, isoniazid, hydralazine) have been shown to worsen the symptoms of SLE.

Scleritis is common in patients with SLE presenting with severe, deep, boring eye pain, lacrimation, photophobia, and congestion of scleral blood vessels. Damage to the lacrimal gland by SLE may cause dry eyes due to poor tear production. Retinopathy, optic neuritis, and cotton wool patches may also occur.

Multiple Sclerosis

The axons of most nerve cells are covered with an insulating layer known as the myelin sheath. Its presence increases the speed of electrical impulses along the axon. Multiple sclerosis (MS) destroys the myelin sheath, causing poor conduction along nerve pathways. Consequently, the organ or tissue innervated by the damaged nerve will not function normally. MS afflicts primarily young adults and is characterized by fluctuating neurological signs and symptoms. Common initial symptoms include weakness of one or more extremities, abnormal sensation (especially over the lower extremities), unilateral visual loss, and incoordination. Symptoms may be bizarre and not easily explained. Exacerbations and remissions that span decades typify the course of MS. The cause of MS is unknown. Treatment is primarily supportive and aimed at stopping progression of the disease.

Multiple sclerosis is a common cause of optic neuritis. This complication usually presents as sudden visual loss in one eye. Pain may or may not be present, and the optic disc is usually swollen. When the appropriate cranial nerves are involved, MS can cause paralysis of the extraocular muscles. Nystagmus is also a common ocular complication.

OphT

Rheumatoid Arthritis

Rheumatoid arthritis (RA) is a chronic inflammatory disease of unknown cause, principally affecting joints and their associated tendons. It is three times more frequent in females, and affects 1% to 2% of the United States population. RA may initially occur in one or many joints and is characterized by morning stiffness, joint pain, easy fatigability, weight loss, and anemia. The most frequently involved joints are those of the hand. It is a multisystem disease and may affect lacrimal and salivary glands, pleura, pericardium, lungs, spleen, bone marrow, and nerves. The course of RA varies with each individual patient—40% have mild disease with long periods of no symptoms, and in 50%, the disease is progressive. Some have a very different course that does not respond to treatment. Drugs such as aspirin, prednisone, gold, and Plaquenil(Sanofi

Winthrop Pharmaceuticals, New York, NY) help reduce pain and inflammation, and in some cases, slow progression of the disease. Physical therapy to preserve muscle strength and joint mobility along with rest during acute episodes is helpful. Juvenile rheumatoid arthritis (JRA) afflicts children and adolescents. Symptoms include fever, progressive arthritis, morning stiffness, rash, generalized lymph node enlargement, and enlargement of the liver and spleen. Treatment for patients with JRA is similar to treatment for adults with RA.

Keratoconjunctivitis sicca is the most common ocular complication of rheumatoid arthritis. It is secondary to lacrimal gland damage, which results in deficient tear production. When RA, keratoconjunctivitis sicca, and xerostomia (insufficient saliva production) occur together, this is known as Sjogren's syndrome. Scleritis and episcleritis are also associated with rheumatoid arthritis. The leading cause of blindness in RA patients is corneal disease caused by scleritis, episcleritis, and keratoconjunctivitis sicca. Uveitis is common in juvenile rheumatoid arthritis.

Plaquenil, a drug used to treat rheumatoid arthritis, can also damage the eye. It is toxic to the retina and causes perimacular pigmentation, retinal edema, and scotomata. These result in decreased visual acuity and color vision. Corneal deposits are also seen. Only 1% of patients taking Plaquenil develop decreased visual acuity, and blindness is very rare. An eye exam is needed every 6 months for adults and every 3 months for children while they are taking the drug. Most toxic effects of Plaquenil are reversible if noticed early and use of the drug is discontinued.

Temporal Arteritis

The temporal artery is a branch of the external carotid artery and can be felt in front of the ear at the temple. Inflammation of the temporal artery is known as temporal arteritis. Arterial inflammation, though, is not limited to the temporal artery, but usually affects many arteries in the head, including those to the eye. Temporal arteritis occurs most often in patients over 60 years of age and is rare in people under 50. Symptoms include pain, tenderness, inflammation over the temporal arteries, pain in the jaw or tongue on chewing or talking, and intermittent visual loss (amaurosis fugax). Sixty to 70% of these patients will also have severe muscle aching and stiffness, fever, weight loss, and depression. These symptoms constitute a co-existing illness known as polymyalgia rheumatica. Temporal arteritis responds favorably to long-term steroid treatment (usually 3 to 6 months of prednisone).

The most severe complication of temporal arteritis is blindness. It occurs in 10% to 50% of untreated patients and is due to ischemic optic neuritis caused by occlusion of arteries supplying the optic nerve. Blindness occurs suddenly and is usually irreversible. High doses of prednisone started early in the course of the disease usually prevent this dreaded complication. Weakness of extraocular muscles is also seen in patients with temporal arteritis.

Chapter 11

Muscle Disorders

KEY POINTS

- Muscular dystrophy is a genetic disease that causes a progressive weakness of muscles.

- Ocular involvement in muscular dystrophy may include weakness of the extraocular muscles (causing diplopia) and of the levator muscle (causing ptosis).

- Muscle weakness is also a hallmark of myasthenia gravis (MG). Ptosis and diplopia are often the initial symptoms.

- If a ptotic lid rises after the patient is injected with Tensilon®, this confirms the diagnosis of MG.

Muscular Dystrophy

Muscular dystrophy refers to a group of inherited diseases that weaken normally developed muscles. The disease usually begins in childhood or adolescence and is characterized by progressive muscle weakness and loss of muscle size. A defective cell membrane is thought to cause the muscle damage seen in this disease. There are a number of different types of muscular dystrophy. They are differentiated by age of onset, patient gender, rate of disease progression, presence or absence of facial involvement, and the muscles initially affected. Duchenne muscular dystrophy is the most severe form, killing most of its victims by age 20. Muscle biopsy and DNA analysis are helpful in diagnosing muscular dystrophy. Since muscular dystrophy is caused by a genetic defect, there is no definitive treatment. Therapy is aimed at keeping the patient mobile and independent as long as possible.

Most eye involvement occurs in two types of muscular dystrophy—oculopharyngeal muscular dystrophy and ocular muscular dystrophy. Oculopharyngeal musculai dystrophy involves the muscles of the eye and pharynx. Patients complain of difficulty swallowing and will present with ptosis or weakness of extraocular muscles. It typically begins after age 30. Ocular muscular dystrophy affects only the eye muscles that cause ptosis and extraocular muscle weakness. It usually presents before age 30.

OphT

Myasthenia Gravis

Motor nerves from the brain to the muscles carry instructions that activate muscle movement. These instructions are relayed to the muscle across a synapse between the axon of the motor neuron and the muscle cells. Acetylcholine is the chemical neurotransmitter that carries the message across the synapse to the muscle. Proteins in the muscle cell membrane receive the acetylcholine and relay the information to the muscle cells, which then carry out the instructions. In myasthenia gravis (MG), the body, for unknown reasons, destroys the receptor proteins in the muscle cell membrane. This disrupts communication between the brain and muscles, resulting in muscle weakness.

Myasthenia gravis usually begins between the ages of 20 and 40. The hallmark of the disease is weak muscles that fatigue easily. Ptosis and diplopia are the usual initial symptoms and are caused by weakness of the extraocular and levator muscles of the eye. The pupil is never involved. MG can involve many muscles, including those of the pharynx (causing problems with swallowing and speaking), respiratory muscles (making breathing difficult), and muscles of the legs and arms. Ten percent of patients with MG also have tumors of the thymus gland. The disease has remissions and exacerbations, usually reaching maximum severity within 1 year.

The Tensilon (ICN Pharmaceuticals, Inc., Costa Mesa, CA) test can be used to diagnose MG. Tensilon is a drug that makes acetylcholine more effective at the nerve-muscle synapse. When given intravenously to a patient with myasthenia gravis, vastly improved muscle strength will be noted within a few minutes. Treatment for MG includes drugs such as pyridostigmine, which can improve muscle strength, and steroids such as prednisone. In some patients, removal of the thymus gland will reverse muscle weakness.

The classic ocular signs of MG are bilateral ptosis (worsens with prolonged upward gaze) and double vision. Ninety percent of patients with generalized MG have eye involvement, while in 20% of patients only the eyes are affected. The diagnosis of MG is confirmed with improvement of ocular muscle function after giving Tensilon (Tensilon test).

Chapter 12

Blood Dyscrasias

KEY POINTS

- The ocular effects of leukemia are caused by the infiltration of abnormal white blood cells into the tissue.

- In the eye, leukemia may cause optic nerve compression and elevated intraocular pressure.

- The ocular effects of anemia can include pale conjunctiva, retinal hemorrhage, cotton wool spots, and hard exudates.

- Ocular problems in sickle cell disease are due to blockage of small arteries by sickled red blood cells.

- In the eye, sickle cell disease may cause neovascularization, vitreous hemorrhage, and retinal detachment.

Blood dyscrasia is a general term used to describe any disease or abnormal condition of the blood. The following sections will discuss three blood dyscrasias—leukemia, anemia, and sickle cell anemia.

Leukemia

Leukemia is a form of cancer that causes large numbers of abnormal white blood cells to be produced by the bone marrow. Normal cells such as platelets, red blood cells, and other white blood cells are crowded out. In most patients, death results from the loss of these normal cells (ie, bleeding from lack of platelets, infection due to lack of effective white blood cells, or anemia due to lack of red blood cells). The symptoms of leukemia include chronic fatigue, reduced exercise tolerance, anemia, fever, bruising, weight loss, enlargement of liver and spleen, and elevated white blood count. Leukemia is the most common form of cancer in children.

There are two categories of white blood cells made in the bone marrow: lymphoid and myeloid. These two categories form the basis for categorizing leukemias. Leukemias affecting lymphoid cells are termed lymphocytic. Those involving myeloid cells are called myelogenous or non-lymphocytic. Further, depending on the speed of disease progression, leukemias can be either acute or chronic.

Acute leukemias make up 10% of all human cancers and are the leading cause of death due to cancer in adults under 35 years of age. Acute non-lymphocytic leukemias make up 80% of acute leukemias, and acute lymphocytic leukemias are responsible for the remainder. Most childhood leukemias are of the latter type. Fortunately, survival rates for acute lymphocytic leukemia can be as high as 80%.

Chronic myelogenous leukemia most often affects people in their 30s, and accounts for 20% of all leukemias in the United States. Chronic lymphocytic leukemia is the most common type of leukemia in western countries and is a disease of people over 50.

Leukemia's ocular effects are due to infiltration of eye tissues by abnormal white blood cells. Any tissue of the eye can be affected, but the choroid and retina are most commonly involved. Optic nerve compression by leukemic cells can threaten vision and require immediate radiation treatment to prevent blindness. Leukemia cells in the vitreous may clog the trabecular meshwork, resulting in elevated intraocular pressure.

Anemia

Anemia occurs when the blood hemoglobin concentration falls below normal range (13 grams in men and 12 grams in nonpregnant women). Symptoms and signs of anemia include fatigue, weakness, shortness of breath on exertion, dizziness, rapid pulse, and pallor of conjunctiva and nail beds.

Red blood cells, where hemoglobin is stored, go through several forms from the time they are "birthed" in the bone marrow until their release in the blood stream as mature cells. The reticulocyte is one form along this path. The percentage of reticulocytes in the blood can be used to measure how fast the bone marrow is making red blood cells. The higher the percentage of reticulocytes, the faster the bone marrow is working. Normally, reticulocytes make up .5% to 2.5% of total red blood cells. The reticulocyte count can be used to classify anemias (Table 12-1).

There are two categories of anemia—those with low or normal reticulocyte counts and those with elevated reticulocyte counts. Each category is further subdivided by red blood cell size.

Paleness of the conjunctiva is commonly seen with anemia and is one of the clinical signs indicating its presence. Retinal hemorrhages, cotton wool spots, and hard exudates, though, are the most common ocular changes seen in anemia.

Table 12-1.
Classes of Anemia

I. Anemias with low or normal reticulocyte counts
    A. Microcytic (red blood cells are smaller than normal)—iron deficiency, some hereditary disorders
    B. Macrocytic (red blood cells are larger than normal)—vitamin B-12 and folate deficiency, chronic liver disease
    C. Normocytic (red blood cells are normal size)—chronic disease such as cancer
II. Anemias with high reticulocyte counts
    A. Microcytic—hemoglobin abnormalities, intravascular destruction of red blood cells
    B. Macrocytic—removal of spleen
    C. Normocytic—acute blood loss or destruction of blood cells (hemolysis)

Sickle Cell Anemia

Sickle cell anemia is an inherited disease affecting 2% of the African-American population. Victims of this disease carry a genetic defect that produces abnormal hemoglobin molecules in their red blood cells. In the presence of low oxygen levels, the red blood cells deform and become shaped like sickles. This distinctive cell shape gives the disease its name. Because of their abnormal shape, these sickled cells cannot pass through small blood vessels. Consequently, the cells block the vessels, depriving the surrounding tissues of needed oxygen and nutrients. This process causes bouts of pain, or crises, which characterize the disorder. The pain of a crisis can occur anywhere in the body, but is most common in the extremities, chest, and back. Pain is typically very severe and requires large doses of strong pain medicine for relief.

Blockage of blood vessels can also damage organs such as the skin, bone, liver, kidney, heart, and lung. Sickle cell patients have less than adequate immune systems, which increases the frequency and severity of infections. All patients have a chronic anemia due to destruction of red blood cells. There is no cure for sickle cell anemia; the goal of treatment is improving the quality and length of life.

Ocular problems in sickle cell disease are also due to blockage of small arteries by sickled red blood cells. Sickle cell retinopathy results when retinal vessels are blocked. This usually begins in the peripheral retina and can progress to new blood vessel formation, hemorrhage into the vitreous, and retinal detachment. Less frequently seen changes include lid edema and iris atrophy.

Chapter 13

Age-Related Disorders

OphMT

KEY POINTS

- Ninety percent of cataracts are due to the normal aging process of the lens.

- There is an increased incidence of chronic open-angle glaucoma and macular degeneration after age 40.

- Loss of hydration can lead to dry eye and loss of muscle tone to disorders of lid position.

- Oxygen use in premature infants can damage the retina, causing retinopathy of prematurity (ROP).

- The retinal damage of ROP is caused by blocked development of the retinal blood vessels. Blindness may result.

Aging

Growing older involves many changes. Physiological capabilities decrease, and a person becomes increasingly more vulnerable to disease. Death also becomes a more real possibility. We age in two ways: chronologically (the number of years we live), and physiologically (the way our body functions).

There has been little change in maximum life span (100 to 120 years) since ancient times. The average life span, however, has significantly increased since the beginning of this century. In 1900, the average person died in their late 40s. Today, it is the norm for people to live into their eighth decade. On average, women live 7 years longer than men.

Physiological aging is characterized by a general slow down and break down in bodily organ function. Below is a list of aging's effects on different areas of the body.

- Immune system—decreased ability to fight infection
- Central nervous system—decreased number of neurons, causing gradual loss of short-term memory, increase in reaction time, and increase in time needed to learn new information
- Cardiovascular system—impaired ability to respond to demands (ie, during exercise)
- Respiratory system—decreased efficiency and exercise tolerance; decreased ability to smell
- Gastrointestinal system—decreased taste, increased constipation
- Musculoskeletal system—breakdown of joints, loss of bone density, and loss of muscle mass
- Reproductive system—decreased sexual responsiveness and reproductive capacity
- Skin—wrinkling and decreased sweating
- Ears—decreased ability to hear high-pitched sounds

Several eye problems are related to aging. Ninety percent of cataracts are due to the normal aging process of the lens. Loss of accommodation also occurs for the same reason. Chronic open-angle glaucoma and macular degeneration become much more common as age increases. Decreased tear production can lead to dry eyes and its associated complications. Loss of skin and muscle function in and around the lid causes disorders such as entropion, ectropion, and dermatochalasis. Extraocular muscle dysfunction may cause deficiencies in upward gaze and convergence.

Prematurity

Respiratory Distress Syndrome (Hyaline Membrane Disease)

Respiratory distress syndrome (RDS) is one of the leading causes of death in premature infants. Seventy percent of infants born before 28 weeks of gestation have this disorder and are the most likely to die from it. RDS occurs when a child is forced to breathe air before his or her lungs are mature enough to do so. Lack of surfactant, a chemical that helps keep air passages open, is the primary cause of this disorder. Because normal ventilation requires surfactant, victims of RDS develop difficulty breathing in the first few hours after birth. Survival frequently requires the use of oxygen and mechanical ventilation. The recently developed ability to replace surfactant has significantly improved outcomes in these infants.

Retinopathy of Prematurity (ROP)

Babies born prematurely often need oxygen to prevent death or brain damage. Unfortunately, in the 1950s, oxygen use in these infants was also shown to damage the retina (retinopathy of prematurity). This entity was at one time the leading cause of blindness in children. Today, 500 children are blinded by ROP each year.

Supplemental oxygen given to the premature infant can block the development of retinal blood vessels. The more premature the baby, the greater the risk that this will occur. Once set in motion, this process can lead to retinal scarring, retinal detachment, and blindness.

Two things put infants at high risk of developing retinopathy of prematurity—receiving supplemental oxygen in the first 7 days of life and weighing less than 1250 grams at birth. Retinal examinations on these children should begin at 4 to 6 weeks of age and be repeated every 2 to 3 weeks thereafter.

Mild forms of ROP may resolve without treatment and have minimal effect on vision. In other cases, cryotherapy or laser treatment can significantly improve outcomes in these children.

Chapter 14

Environmental Disorders

KEY POINTS

- The most severe ocular effects of malnutrition are night blindness, retinopathy, and corneal ulceration/necrosis.

- Ocular effects of alcoholism can include visual field defects, nerve palsies, optic atrophy, alcohol amblyopia, decreased color perception, and cataracts.

- The most common ocular effect of smoking is chronic conjunctival irritation caused by smoke exposure.

- Retinal and vitreal hemorrhages due to head trauma are the most common ocular signs of child abuse.

Malnutrition

Malnutrition occurs when insufficient protein or calories are present to meet bodily needs. This causes impairment of the body's normal physiologic processes. Malnutrition due to calorie deficiency is called marasmus, while that due to protein deficiency is called kwashiorkor. The more current designation is protein calorie malnutrition (PCM) or protein energy malnutrition (PEM), respectively.

There are several causes of PEM, the most common being inadequate protein or calorie intake. Increased nutritional needs and loss of nutrients during disease can result in insufficient nourishment to meet bodily demands. Poor protein quality may also precipitate PEM.

In the United States, the highest incidence of malnutrition occurs among institutionalized senior citizens and children of the poor. Preschool children are most susceptible to malnutrition because they have to depend on others for their intake, and their protein and energy demands are greater per unit of weight than adults. Worldwide, gastrointestinal infections are a major cause of malnutrition in infants and children.

Weight loss and loss of subcutaneous fat are the most common signs of malnutrition in adults. In children, stunted physical development, delayed puberty, and poor mental and social maturation are the result.

Body weight can be used to classify PEM in adults. An unintentional weight loss of less than 10% is termed mild PEM. Moderate PEM is an unintentional weight loss of 10% to 20%, while severe PEM occurs with an unintentional weight loss of greater than 20%.

The effects of malnutrition on the body include the following:
- Gastrointestinal—atrophy, loss of ability to absorb nutrients
- Immune system—impaired, increased risk of infection
- Endocrine—decreased thyroid function, infertility, cessation of menses
- Cardiovascular—heart muscle atrophy, conduction system abnormalities
- Respiratory—atrophy of respiratory muscles (impairs breathing)

The most common (and severe) ocular effects of malnutrition are related to vitamin A deficiency. Both protein and calorie malnutrition limit the availability and use of vitamin A in the body. Two eye-related disorders characterize vitamin A deficiency. Xerophthalmia refers to a broad range of ocular problems caused by vitamin A deficiency including night blindness, retinopathy, and corneal ulceration. Keratomalacia is thought to be the final stage of xerophthalmia and causes corneal necrosis.

Alcoholism

Alcoholism, as defined by the National Council on Alcoholism and Drug Dependence, is a primary chronic disease with genetic, psychosocial, and environmental factors influencing its development and manifestations. The condition is often progressive and fatal. It is characterized by impaired control of drinking, preoccupation with alcohol, use of alcohol despite adverse consequences, and distortions in thinking (most notably denial). Each of these symptoms may be continuous or periodic. An estimated 10.5 million Americans are alcoholics. Risk factors for developing alcoholism include a family history of alcoholism, history of other drug abuse, onset of drinking at an early age, behavioral problems early in life, and exposure to social or occupational situations where alcohol is readily available and the pressure to drink is strong. Insomnia, depression, nightmares, poor memory, nervousness, abdominal complaints, sexual problems, and evidence of repeated injury are symptoms of alcoholism. The diagnosis of alcoholism can be made when the following four elements are present for at least 1 month: loss of ability to control the drinking, adverse outcome(s) resulting from drinking, evidence of addiction to alcohol, and drinking in quantities or frequency that are considered excessive.

The consequences of alcoholism are many and severe. Alcohol use is involved in 50% of all motor vehicle accident fatalities, 67% of all murders, and 33% of suicides. Alcoholism can result in damage to the brain, liver, pancreas, gastrointestinal tract, and heart. Fetal alcohol syndrome afflicts many infants born to alcoholic mothers. Characteristics of these children include facial abnormalities, mental retardation, low birth weight and length, and deformities of the cardiovascular and skeletal systems.

The primary treatment for alcoholism is professional counseling and involvement in support groups such as Alcoholics Anonymous. Antabuse (Wyeth Ayerst Laboratories, Philadelphia) is a drug used to discourage alcohol ingestion. Any alcohol taken while on this drug causes a very uncomfortable physical reaction. This helps the alcoholic resist the urge to drink.

Ocular effects of alcoholism include visual field defects, nerve palsies, optic atrophy, vision loss in one eye (alcohol amblyopia), decreased color perception, and cataracts. Optic neuritis can occur as a side effect of Antabuse treatment. Fetal alcohol syndrome victims may present with short palpebral fissures, strabismus, ptosis, and pale optic discs.

Cigarette Smoking

Smoking is the most common cause of preventable disease, as well as the largest single health risk in the United States. Approximately 30% of the US population smokes, and 1 million children and teenagers start smoking every year.

More than 4000 substances have been identified in cigarette smoke. The most widely known of these is the toxic drug nicotine. Nicotine is a stimulant to the cardiovascular system causing increased heart rate and blood pressure, irritability of heart muscle, and constriction of blood vessels. It is believed to be responsible for the addictive nature of cigarette smoking. In the addicted individual, withdrawal of nicotine causes anger, anxiety, hunger, impatience, restlessness, difficulty concentrating, and craving for cigarettes. Symptoms are worst at 1 to 2 days and usually resolve in 3 to 4 weeks, but may last for an extended period of time. Other significant components of cigarette smoke include carbon dioxide (which interferes with the body's ability to use and transport oxygen), cancer causing chemicals (such as tar, hydrocarbons, hydrazine, vinyl chloride), and substances that irritate the bronchial system and interfere with the lung's ability to clear secretions (acetaldehyde, formaldehyde, and ammonia).

A number of negative physical consequences have been associated with cigarette smoking. Men who smoke have a 70% higher death rate than non-smoking men. The same holds true for women smokers but to a lesser degree. Female smokers, on average, go through menopause sooner than non-smokers. Smokers have decreased exercise performance and impaired immune systems. There is a strong association between smoking and atherosclerotic cardiovascular disease (heart attacks and stroke), cancer (responsible for 30% of all cancer deaths), and chronic obstructive lung disease (chronic bronchitis and emphysema). Smoking during pregnancy increases the risk of spontaneous abortion, fetal death, and sudden infant death syndrome. Gastrointestinal ulcer disease is also more common in smokers. Passive smoke inhalation increases the risk of early death in adults and the risk of lung infections and ear problems in children.

The most common ocular effect of smoking is chronic conjunctival irritation caused by smoke exposure. Smoking also increases the risk of nuclear sclerotic cataracts and age-related macular degeneration, and optic nerve damage is more severe in glaucoma patients who smoke. Nystagmus, prolonged postoperative wound healing, and optic neuropathy (tobacco-alcohol amblyopia) have also been associated with cigarette smoking.

Child Abuse

Legally defined, child abuse is "the physical or mental injury, sexual abuse, negligent treatment, or maltreatment of a child under the age of 18 by a person who is responsible for the child's welfare under circumstances which indicate that the child's health or welfare is harmed or threatened thereby" (Child Abuse Prevention and Treatment Act of 1974).

Until the early 1960s the medical community was largely uninformed about the presentation and frequency of child abuse. This changed in 1962 when CH Kempe first used the term "battered child syndrome," and brought the problem into prominence in both medical and public arenas. The enactment of laws in all states making it mandatory for healthcare professionals to report suspected cases of child abuse resulted from Kempe's work.

The majority of abused children are under 4 years of age. Certain children are at greater risk of being abused. These include unwanted children of accidental or illegitimate pregnancies, children who are the opposite sex of what a parent wanted, children born during periods of crisis, children resulting from a relationship other than the present one (ie, stepchildren), and children who are difficult to care for (ie, excessive crying or abnormal sleep patterns).

Child abuse can be either active or passive. Withholding basic needs constitutes passive abuse. This would include denial of proper food, medical care, or nurture. If negligence begins in infancy, a child will fail to develop normally. These children appear wide-eyed and cautious, avoid eye contact and physical affection, prefer inanimate objects over animate objects, are difficult to console, and spend a lot of time with their hands in their mouths. Most are malnourished and small for their age. Termed "failure to thrive," these symptoms are usually seen in children under 3 years of age.

Active abuse occurs when a child is treated in an inappropriate way. Physical and sexual abuse are the two major forms of active abuse.

Physical abuse (non-accidental trauma) takes many forms. Examples include beatings, burns, poisoning, and murder. Two-thirds of physical abuse victims are under the age of 3, and 95% are abused by their parents. Physically abused children who are returned to their parents without intervention are killed in 5% to 10% of cases, and 35% to 50% are seriously re-injured. This is why recognition and reporting of an abusive situation is so important.

Several characteristics of an incident make abuse more likely. A suspicious injury is one that is unlikely to occur in the child's age group, such as leg burns from hot water immersion on a child too young to walk. The caretaker's description of the incident may be inconsistent with the child's injuries, and multiple injuries may be present. Facts about the incident can change, and the child's description of what happened is different from the caretaker's. Many times there is a delay in seeking medical attention.

The most common physical manifestation of abuse is bruising. In many cases, bruising from abuse can be differentiated from bruising due to other causes. Accidental bruising is usually seen over bony protrusions such as knees, chin, elbows, or forehead. Bruising due to abuse commonly occurs over buttocks, lower back, genitals, lower thighs, cheeks, earlobes, or neck, and will be shaped like the instrument used to inflict it.

Another frequently seen result of physical abuse is fractures. Fractures seen in children under 1 year of age frequently result from abuse. The most common fractures seen in abused children are rib fractures.

A third often seen presentation of abuse is intracranial hemorrhage. This is caused by direct blows to the head or by shaken baby syndrome. Shaken baby syndrome occurs when vigorous shaking of a child (usually under 15 months of age) causes bruising of and bleeding into the brain. Fifteen percent of these children die, and 50% have significant brain damage.

Sexual abuse usually occurs in the 2 to 6 and 12 to 16 age groups. The majority of abusers are known by or are members of the child's family. It is estimated that 25% to 36% of women and 10% to 23% of men are sexually abused at some point in their lives. Thirty to 50% of all child abuse cases are sexual abuse.

Sexually abused children often present with genitourinary tract problems such as vaginal discharge, vaginal bleeding, pain on urination, urinary tract infections, or discharge from the urethra. These symptoms may indicate the presence of a sexually transmitted disease such as gonorrhea, syphilis, or chlamydia. Any child with a sexually transmitted disease is sexually abused until proven otherwise. Behavioral disturbances, sexually oriented or provocative behavior, and nightmares are commonly seen in the sexually abused. These children are often victims of physical abuse as well. Sexually abused children usually will not reveal abuse until some time after the incident.

The ocular problems of child abuse are primarily due to physical abuse. Retinal and vitreal hemorrhages due to head trauma are the most common ocular signs. These may be present when no other indication of abuse is evident. One or both eyes may be involved. Retinal scarring, optic atrophy, and blindness can result. Thus, ophthalmoscopy is mandatory in any suspected case of child abuse. Other ocular consequences of abuse include periorbital bruising and swelling, orbital fractures, subconjunctival hemorrhage, hyphema, dislocated lens, and retinal detachment.

Chapter 15

Genetic Disorders

OphMT

KEY POINTS

- Albinism is a genetic defect in which the person's body produces no melanin (pigment).

- Ocular effects of albinism include a blue-gray to pink iris, nystagmus, decreased visual acuity, strabismus, and photophobia.

- Down syndrome occurs when there are three number 21 chromosomes (instead of two).

- Ocular effects of Down syndrome include short, slanted palpebral fissure, epicanthal folds, strabismus, nystagmus, myopia, and cataracts.

Albinism

Melanin, a pigment produced by cells called melanocytes, is the main cause of color in the skin, hair, and eyes (iris and retina). In addition to its cosmetic effects, melanin has three other benefits:

- it helps prevent light damage to the skin
- it blocks light from passing through the iris to the retina
- it absorbs extraneous light striking the retina that could interfere with visual acuity.

Due to a genetic defect, some people have melanocytes that produce no melanin. Consequently, their skin, hair, or eyes have little or no color. This condition is called albinism. Approximately one in 30,000 people in the United States are afflicted with this disorder.

There are three forms of albinism—oculocutaneous, ocular, and partial albinism.

Oculocutaneous albinism involves pigment loss in both skin and eyes, while ocular albinism affects only the eyes. Partial albinism does not affect the eyes, and skin depigmentation is localized to the forehead, anterior scalp (typically there is white lock of hair near their forehead), anterior trunk, elbows, or knees.

Albinism's effects on the eye are the same from patient to patient. They include nystagmus, decreased visual acuity, loss of pigment in the iris and retina (the iris is usually blue-gray to pink), an underdeveloped macula (the main cause of decreased visual acuity), strabismus, and photophobia. Additionally, the optic nerve fibers do not cross normally at the optic chiasm, causing absence of binocular vision.

Albinism has three major consequences. First, due to a lack of melanin's protective effects on the skin there is an increased incidence of skin cancer. Second, decreased visual acuity and ultimately blindness create a significant handicap. Third, the impact of the above can result in substantial psychological problems.

Down Syndrome

Down syndrome was first described in 1866 by Dr. Langdon Down, an English physician. Its cause, however, was not determined until 1959 by a group of French scientists.

A normal human has 23 pairs of chromosomes, which are numbered 1 through 22 (the 23rd pair is the sex chromosomes). Instead of the usual two chromosomes, patients with Down syndrome have three number 21 chromosomes. This is why trisomy 21 is an alternate name for Down syndrome. It is the most common chromosomal disorder observed in the newborn period, occurring once in every 600 to 800 births. Half of all Down syndrome children are born to women over 35 years of age.

Down syndrome causes several abnormalities. The physical appearance is characteristically a flat face, short broad hands, and short stature. Their birth weight is usually below average, and varying degrees of mental retardation will be present. (Down syndrome is the most common cause of mental retardation.) Other problems include decreased muscle tone, deformities of the pelvis, cardiac malformations (30% to 60%), a high-arched palate, and intestinal deformities. Immune system abnormalities can also occur, resulting in a high incidence of leukemia and infections (primarily ear, throat, and sinus infections).

There are several ocular manifestations of Down syndrome. The palpebral fissures are slanted upward and about 7 mm shorter than normal. Epicanthal folds give a hooded appearance to the eyes. White to light yellow spots at the periphery of the iris (Brushfield spots) are frequently seen. There is a high incidence of eyelid infections, and 20% to 40% of patients have strabismus. Horizontal nystagmus, keratoconus, cataracts, myopia, and astigmatism are also commonly seen in patients with Down syndrome.

Chapter 16

Neoplastic Disorders

KEY POINTS

- Cancer from other areas of the body can metastasize to the eye; the uvea is the most common site.

- Non-Hodgkin's lymphoma (NHL) is a cancer of the lymph tissue.

- Ocular involvement in NHL is rare but can include the orbit, lacrimal gland, and conjunctiva.

Metastatic Cancer

Metastatic is a cancer that has spread from one organ to another that is not directly connected to it. For example, if lung cancer spreads to the brain, it is considered metastatic lung cancer since the lungs and brain are not directly connected.

Cancers that metastasize to the eye include:

- Orbit—breast, lung, prostate, and melanoma
- Uvea (most common site of metastasis)—breast, lung, gastrointestinal tract, kidney, and thyroid
- Eyelid—breast, lung, and cutaneous melanoma
- Conjunctiva—leukemia and lymphoma

Non-Hodgkin's Lymphoma

Lymph tissues help protect the body from infection by filtering the blood and removing infectious agents. These tissues are located throughout the body in small clumps called nodes. They are often enlarged during infections and are sometimes referred to as enlarged "glands." Lymph tissue is also found in the tonsils and spleen.

Cancers that develop in lymph tissue are called lymphomas. They are the sixth most common type of cancer in the United States. There are two types of lymphoma: Hodgkin's lymphoma and non-Hodgkin's lymphoma (NHL). Forty-seven thousand new cases of lymphoma are discovered each year, 85% being non-Hodgkin's lymphoma. Hodgkin's lymphoma seldom involves the eye and will not be discussed.

Patients who contract NHL are typically in their 40s or 50s. The symptoms of NHL are not dramatic, which can result in a 1- to 2-year delay in diagnosis. Persistent painless enlargement of lymph nodes in peripheral areas of the body (ie, where they can be felt) is the most common initial finding in these patients. Enlarged lymph nodes inside the chest occur in 20% of patients, causing cough, chest pain, or an abnormal chest x-ray. Abdominal involvement may precipitate abdominal pain or obstruction of the intestinal tract. More aggressive forms of NHL can invade the brain or bone marrow. Other symptoms of non-Hodgkin's lymphoma, though not typical, include fever, night sweats, and weight loss. While the cause of this disease is still in doubt, viral infection and genetic inheritance are the two most common theories. The diagnosis of NHL is made by taking a piece (biopsy) of an involved lymph node and examining it under a microscope. The mainstay of treatment is chemotherapy, though radiation is effective in some cases. Five-year survival rates vary from 20% to 70%.

Ocular manifestations of NHL occur in only 1% to 2% of cases. It is, however, one of the few life-threatening diseases that an ophthalmologist is likely to diagnose. The most commonly involved site is the orbit, resulting in proptosis and interference with ocular movement. The lacrimal gland is affected in 30% of cases. NHL can also infiltrate the conjunctiva, causing salmon or pink-colored growths.

Chapter 17

Other Disorders

KEY POINTS

- Ocular effects of gout can include redness, elevated intraocular pressure, and uric acid crystals in the cornea or sclera.

- Bilateral anterior uveitis is the most common ocular effect of sarcoidosis.

- Ocular changes in chronic obstructive pulmonary disease are caused by low blood oxygen levels and include dilation of retinal blood vessels.

- Ocular changes during a normal pregnancy may include minor refractive shifts, a drop in intraocular pressure, and mild ptosis.

Gout

Purine is an important chemical that is produced by the body and is also present in the foods we eat (ie, liver, kidney, and anchovies). When the body metabolizes purine, uric acid is produced. Normally, uric acid is removed from the body via the kidneys and intestines. When these processes malfunction, uric acid accumulates in the blood and body tissues, causing gout. Gout is an inflammatory disease caused by deposition of uric acid crystals in and around joints. There are two kinds of gout—primary gout and secondary gout.

Primary gout results from an inherited tendency to overproduce or underexcrete uric acid. This causes the high blood uric acid level, which is characteristic of gout. Secondary gout is the result of other diseases or drug therapy. For example, cancer can cause an over-production of uric acid, and kidney disease, aspirin, alcohol, lead poisoning, and diuretics prevent proper excretion of uric acid in the urine.

Gout usually affects men 40 to 60 years old and postmenopausal women. Acute recurring attacks of severe joint pain are typical of gout. The most commonly involved area is the first joint of the big toe. The affected joints are reddened and swollen, and even light touch can cause severe discomfort. Overindulgence in food and alcohol, infection, surgery, and emotional stress have all been known to precipitate an acute gouty attack. The best way to diagnose gout is to take a sample of fluid from an involved joint and examine it for uric acid crystals. If crystals are found, then gout is present. Elevated blood levels of uric acid are also seen in most cases of gout. In early gout, there may be no symptoms between acute attacks. As gout progresses, though, chronic pain, swelling, and deformity in multiple joints can occur. This may lead to significant disability. In advanced disease, tophi (large deposits of uric acid) can appear in and around joints, causing deformity. Gout can also cause renal disease as well as kidney stones.

Acute attacks of gout are treated with pain medicine and anti-inflammatory drugs like cortisone and indomethacin. Between attacks, blood levels of uric acid are controlled with two types of drugs—allopurinal (which blocks production of uric acid), and probenecid and sulfinpyrazone (which increase excretion of uric acid in the urine).

Traditionally, gout has been thought to cause uveitis. However, recent studies fail to show this to be a frequent occurrence. Crystals of uric acid in the cornea (fine, golden yellow, and shiny) or on the sclera are sometimes seen with the slit lamp. Gout has also been associated with elevated intraocular pressure and red eyes (due to scleritis, episcleritis, and conjunctivitis).

Sarcoidosis

Sarcoidosis is a disease of unknown cause that affects many areas of the body. Its characteristic finding is small tumors (called granulomas) that invade and damage bodily organs. Victims of the disease are usually in their 20s or 30s, and are most often African-American, Puerto Rican, or Scandinavian. General symptoms include fatigue, weight loss, fever, and malaise. Shortness of breath, dry cough, and chest pain occur when the lungs are involved (90% of patients). Blood calcium levels are frequently elevated at some point during the course of the illness. Other findings include enlargement of lymph nodes, liver, and spleen, an abnormal heart beat, facial nerve weakness, and arthritis. Twenty percent of patients with sarcoidosis will have no symptoms but will have findings on chest x-ray that suggests the diagnosis.

Most victims of sarcoidosis (60%) get well over several years without treatment. Twenty to 25% will have eye involvement or significant organ damage that require steroid treatment. The remainder will have a chronic and sometimes progressive form of the disease.

Bilateral anterior uveitis is the most common effect of sarcoidosis on the eye. All patients suspected of having sarcoidosis should have a careful slit lamp examination to rule out uveitis. Granulomas may be seen on the iris or eyelids and may cause painless enlargement of the lacrimal gland. The optic nerve is commonly involved, resulting in optic neuritis or atrophy and other abnormalities.

Chronic Obstructive Pulmonary Disease

As the name suggests, chronic obstructive pulmonary disease (COPD) is a long-term blockage of the airways in the lung. Damage to the lungs caused by cigarette smoking, air pollution, occupational exposure to irritating substances, or infection is the underlying cause of COPD.

The narrowed breathing passages in this disease inhibit the patient's ability to move air in and out of the lungs. Because airflow is restricted, blood levels of oxygen are usually lower than normal. The combination of low blood oxygen levels and lung damage increases blood pressure in the lungs. This adds an additional strain on the heart that can cause heart failure (cor pulmonale). There are two disease processes involved in most COPD: chronic bronchitis and emphysema.

Chronic bronchitis is defined as excessive airway mucous production causing a cough 3 months per year for 2 consecutive years. In addition, the airway walls become thickened and scarred, which further restricts airflow. Symptoms include wheezing, shortness of breath, and excessive coughing with copious sputum production. These patients are usually overweight and have a bluish color (cyanosis) due to lack of oxygen. For this reason, they are called "blue bloaters."

Emphysema, on the other hand, results from distention of alveoli and surrounding airways and destruction of alveolar walls. This, along with airway obstruction, compromises the lung's ability to absorb oxygen. Symptoms include shortness of breath, wheezing, and cough with little mucous production. These patients are usually underweight and have a pinkish coloration. They are labeled "pink puffers."

There are five elements of COPD treatment:
1. Remove the cause (ie, stop smoking)
2. Drugs to dilate the airway
3. Steroids to reduce inflammation
4. Supplemental oxygen
5. Aggressive treatment of infections

Ocular changes in COPD are caused by low blood oxygen levels. The retinal and conjunctival blood vessels become darker in color, and retinal arteries and veins dilate. With severe lung disease, retinal hemorrhages with macular and optic disc edema may occur.

Eye Changes During Normal Pregnancy

Minor refractive shifts and difficulty with accommodation may occur in the later stages of pregnancy. These changes are probably due to increased fluid content in the cornea or lens caused by the hormone progesterone. New refractions or contact lens fittings should be deferred until several weeks after pregnancy has ended.

Intraocular pressure may drop during the second half of pregnancy. The change, however, is temporary, and by 2 months after delivery it has usually returned to normal.

Occasionally, mild ptosis will develop during pregnancy. This often resolves after delivery, though occasionally levator surgery is needed.

Pregnancy-induced increases in melanocyte stimulating hormone can cause hyperpigmentation of the eyelids.

In women with longstanding diabetes, retinopathy may develop or worsen during pregnancy. Some changes resolve spontaneously after birth, but others require laser therapy.

Bibliography

Baker RC. *Handbook of Pediatric Primary Care*. Boston, Mass: Little, Brown and Company; 1996.

Basmajian JV. *Primary Anatomy*. Baltimore, Md: Williams and Wilkins; 1982.

Basmajian JV, Slonecker CE. *Grant's Method of Anatomy: A Clinical Problem Solving Approach*. Baltimore, Md: Williams and Wilkins; 1989.

Behman RE, Kliegman RM, Arvin AM, Nelson WE. *Nelson Textbook of Pediatrics*. Philadelphia, Pa: WB Saunders Co; 1996.

Berne RM, Levy MN. *Principles of Physiology*. St. Louis, Mo: Mosby; 1996.

Christensen JB. *Synopsis of Gross Anatomy*. Philadelphia, Pa: JB Lippincott Company; 1988.

Crouch JE. *Essential Human Anatomy*. Philadelphia, Pa: Lea and Febiger; 1982.

Dale DC, Federman DD. *Scientific American Medicine*. New York, NY: Scientific American, Inc; 1997.

Dornbrand L, Hoole AJ, Pickard CG. *Manual of Clinical Problems in Adult Ambulatory Care*. Boston, Mass: Little, Brown and Company; 1992.

Ewald GA, McKenzie CR. *Manual of Medical Therapeutics*. Boston, Mass: Little, Brown and Company; 1995.

Gatz AJ. *Manter's Essentials of Clinical Neuroanatomy and Neurophysiology*. Philadelphia, Pa: FA Davis Company; 1970.

Gold DH, Weingeist TA. *The Eye in Systemic Disease*. Philadelphia, Pa: JB Lippincott; 1990.

Isselbacher KJ, Braunwald E, Wilson JD, Martin JB, Fauci AS, Kasper DL. *Harrison's Principles of Internal Medicine*. New York, NY: McGraw-Hill; 1995.

Lindsay DT. *Functional Human Anatomy*. St. Louis, Mo: Mosby; 1996.

Mazza JJ. *Manual of Clinical Hematology*. Boston, Mass: Little, Brown and Company; 1995.

McMinn RH, Gaddum-Rosse P, Thutching R, Logan BM. *McMinn's Functional and Clinical Anatomy*. London, England: Mosby;1995.

Oski FA, Deangelis CD, Feigin RD, McMullan JA, Warshaw JB. *Principles and Practice of Pediatrics*. Philadelphia, Pa: JB Lippincott; 1994.

Reese RE, Betts RF. *A Practical Approach to Infectious Disease*. Boston, Mass: Little, Brown and Company; 1996.

Romanes FJ. *Cunningham's Textbook of Anatomy*. Oxford, England: Oxford University Press; 1981.

Rosen P, Doris PE, Barkin RM, Barkin SZ, Markovchick VJ. *Diagnostic Radiology in Emergency Medicine*. St. Louis, Mo: Mosby Yearbook; 1992.

Snell R, Smith M. *Clinical Anatomy for Emergency Medicine*. St. Louis, Mo: Mosby; 1993.

Spence AP, Mason EB. *Human Anatomy and Physiology*. Menlo Park, Calif: Benjamin Cummings Publishing Company, Inc; 1987.

Stewart JV. *Clinical Anatomy and Pathophysiology for Health Professionals*. Miami, Fla: Medmaster, Inc; 1990.

Tasman W, Jaeger EA. *Duane's Ophthalmology*. Philadelphia, Pa: Lippincott Raven; 1997.

Taylor RB. *Manual of Family Practice*. Boston, Mass: Little, Brown and Company; 1997.

Thibodeau GA. *Structure and Function of the Body*. St. Louis, Mo: Mosby Yearbook;1992.

Appendix

Diagnostics

KEY POINTS

- Blood tests that may be indicated in eyecare include complete blood count, blood glucose level, rheumatoid factor, and sedimentation rate.

- X-rays are used to image bony structures.

- Computed tomography uses fanned-out x-rays to create a cross-sectional picture of structures.

- Ultrasound utilizes sound waves to measure or create an image of the eye.

- Magnetic resonance imaging utilizes a magnetic field to create a picture. It is especially useful in imaging soft tissue.

Normal Values of Common Blood Tests

Complete blood count (CBC)—Checks the number of red blood cells, white blood cells, and platelets present in a blood sample. Normal values are:
- White blood cell count: 4300 to 10,800/cu mm
- Platelet count: 150,000 to 350,000/cu mm
- Red cell count
  - Female: 4.2 to 5.4 million/cu mm
  - Male: 4.6 to 6.2 million/cu mm
- Hemoglobin
  - Male: 14 to 17 g/dl
  - Female: 12 to 15 g/dl
- Hematocrit
  - Male: 41% to 50%
  - Female: 36% to 44%

Prothrombin time—Evaluates the blood's ability to clot. A normal value is between 9 and 18 seconds.

Blood glucose level—Used to detect the presence of diabetes and to monitor its treatment. Normal fasting blood glucose level is 60 to 100 mg/dl.

Rheumatoid factor—A test for rheumatoid arthritis. If the patient does not have rheumatoid arthritis, the test will usually be negative.

Erythrocyte sedimentation rate—Indicates the presence and intensity of an inflammatory process such as arthritis or cancer. It is not specific for any one disease. Normal values (Westergren) are:
  - Male: 0 to 13 mm/hour
  - Female: 0 to 20 mm/hour

Creatinine and blood urea nitrogen (BUN)—Both creatinine and BUN are tests of kidney function. Normal values are:
- Creatinine: 0.8 to 1.2 mg/dl
- BUN: 8 to 25 mg/dl

Potassium—3.3 to 4.9 mmol/L
Sodium—135 to 145 mmol/L
Calcium—8.9 to 10.3 mg/dl

X-rays

Wilhelm Conrad Roentgen discovered x-rays in 1895. Because he didn't know what kind of rays they were, he labeled them "x" for unknown. They since have been found to be a type of ionizing radiation. Different types of tissue allow varying amounts of x-rays to pass through. This produces an image of the area being examined, especially bony structures (Figure A-1). By putting photographic film behind the body part being x-rayed, this image is recorded. A doctor can then examine the picture and gather information about a patient's problem. In ophthalmology, an x-ray might be used to identify bone fractures, foreign bodies, and tumors.

Computed Tomography (CT or CAT scan)

The CT scanner uses ionizing radiation to produce an image just like x-rays. Instead of photographic film, electronic radiation detectors are used to capture information. The radiation beam

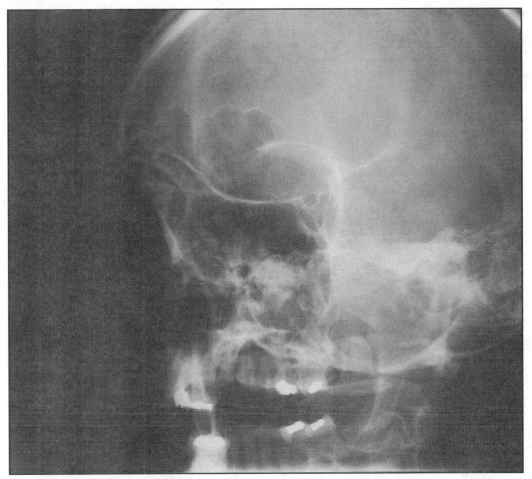

Figure A-1. An x-ray showing the orbits. (Melissa Cabe RT(R) and Jim Ledford, PA-C.)

and sensor rotate around the patient, producing cross-sectional images of the body. These images are displayed on a television monitor and usually printed on normal photographic film (Figure A-2). Dye can be injected as part of the procedure in order to provide contrast on the film. A CT of the head (which includes the orbits) might be ordered to help identify a tumor, fracture, or inflammation.

Ultrasound

Ultrasound uses no radiation. A hand-held instrument transmits sound waves into the body. The structures being examined reflect varying amounts of the sound back to the transmitter. This information is analyzed by a computer, which reconstructs the body parts being "seen" by the ultrasound and displays them on a television monitor. In ophthalmology, an A-scan is used to measure the length of the eye (Figure A-3). A B-scan creates a two-dimensional view of the eye and is used to identify foreign bodies, hemorrhages, tumors, and retinal detachments (Figure A-4).

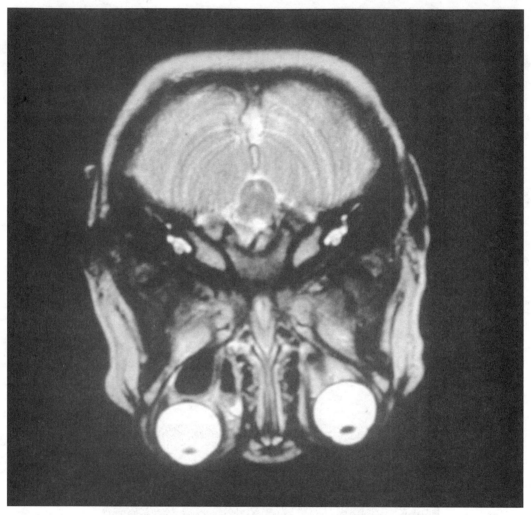

Figure A-2. A CT scan showing the orbits. (Mark Greenwald, University of Tennessee-Memphis.)

Magnetic Resonance Imaging (MRI)

When an MRI scan is done, the patient is put in a strong magnetic field. The tissue to be studied is then bombarded with radio waves. This causes the atoms of the tissue to emit an electronic signal. The signals are captured, and a computer uses them to reconstruct an image of the examined tissue. It is displayed on a television monitor and can be printed on photographic film or stored on computer disk (Figure A-5). MRI scans are especially good for examining soft tissue. In ophthalmology, an MRI might be ordered to better evaluate the patient for swelling, tumors, and nerve conditions. Because the MRI uses a strong magnetic field, any patient with a pacemaker or embedded metal (implants or shrapnel for example) cannot have the test.

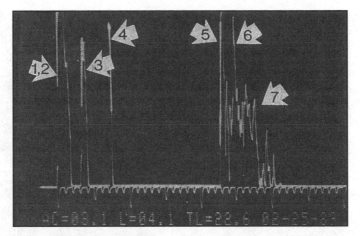

Figure A-3. Typical A-scan for measuring axial length—cornea (1,2), anterior lens (3), posterior lens (4), retina (5), sclera (6), orbital fat (7) (courtesy of Kendall CJ. *Ophthalmic Echography*. Thorofare, NJ: SLACK Incorporated; 1990).

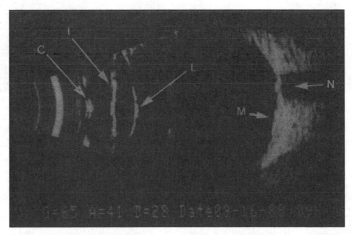

Figure A-4. Typical B-scan—corneal echoes (C), iris (I), posterior lens (L), macula (M), optic nerve (N) (courtesy of Kendall CJ. *Ophthalmic Echography*. Thorofare, NJ: SLACK Incorporated; 1990).

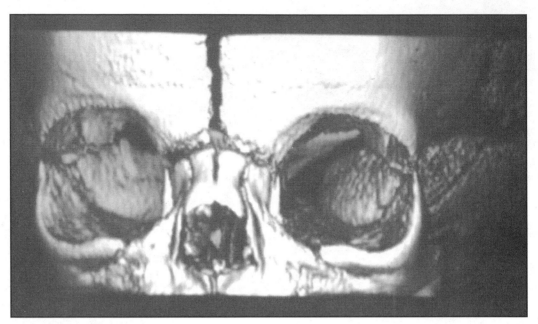

Figure A-5. An MRI showing the orbits. (Mark Greenwald, University of Tennessee-Memphis.)

Index